A FEAST OF INFORMATION—
for people who love to eat but need to know
the calorie count of their meals.

THE BARBARA KRAUS 1985 CALORIE
GUIDE TO BRAND NAMES AND BASIC
FOODS lists thousands of basic and ready-to-eat
foods from appetizers to desserts—carry it to the
supermarket, to the restaurant, to the beach, to
the coffee cart, and on trips.

Flip through these fact-filled pages. Mix, match,
and keep track of calories as they add up. But
remember, strawberry shortcake is fattening any
way you slice it!

The Barbara Kraus
1985 Calorie
Guide to
Brand Names and
Basic Foods

The Barbara Kraus 1985 Calorie Guide to Brand Names and Basic Foods

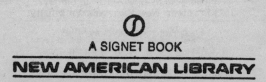

A SIGNET BOOK

NEW AMERICAN LIBRARY

Excerpted from *Dictionary of Calories and Carbohydrates*

*For Frank, Josie, Joey
and Rose Marie Cantasano*

Foreword

The composition of the foods we eat is not static: it changes from time to time. In the case of *brand-name* products, manufacturers alter their recipes to reflect the availability of ingredients, advances in technology, or improvements in formulae. Each year new products appear on the market and some old ones are discontinued.

On the other hand, information on *basic foods* such as meats, vegetables, and fruits may also change as a result of the development of better analytical methods, different growing conditions, or new marketing practices. These changes, however, are usually relatively small as compared with those in manufactured products.

Some differences may be found between the values in this book and those appearing on the product labels. This is usually due to the fact that the Food and Drug Administration permits manufacturers to round the figures reported on labels. The data in this book are reported as calculated without rounding. If large differences between the two sets of values are noted, they may be due to changes in product formulae, and in those cases the label data should be used.

For all these reasons, a book of calorie or nutritive values of foods must be kept up to date by a periodic reviewing and revision of the data presented.

Therefore, this handy calorie counter will provide each year the most current and accurate estimates available. Generous use of this little book will help you and your family to select the right foods and the proper number of calories each member requires to gain, lose, or maintain healthy and attractive weight.

Good eating in 1985! For 1986, we'll pick up the new products, drop any has-beens, and make whatever other changes are necessary.

Barbara Kraus

Why This Book?

Some of the data presented here can be found in more detail in my bestselling *Calories and Carbohydrates*, a dictionary of 8,000 brand names and basic foods. Complete as it is, it is meant to be used as a reference book at home or in the office and not to be squeezed into a suit jacket or evening bag—it's just too big.

Therefore, responding to the need for a portable calorie guide, and one which can reflect food changes often, I have written this smaller and handier version. The selection of material and the additional new entries provide readers with pertinent data on thousands of products that they would prepare at home to take to work, eat in a restaurant or luncheonette, nibble on from the coffee cart, take to the beach, buy in the candy store, etcetera.

For the sake of saving space and providing you with a greater selection of products, I had to make certain compromises: whereas in the giant book there are several physical descriptions of a product, here there is but one.

For Beginners Only

The language of dieting is no more difficult to learn than any other new subject; in many respects, it's much easier, particularly if you restrict your education to clearly defined goals.

For you who never before had the need or the interest in a lesson in weight control, I offer the following elementary introduction, applicable to any diet, self-initiated or suggested by your doctor, nutritionist, or dietician.

A Calorie

An analysis of foods in terms of calories is most often the chosen method to describe the relative energy yielded by foods.

A calorie is a shorthand way to summarize the units of energy contained in any foodstuff or alcoholic beverage, similar to the way a thermometer indicates heat. One pound of fat is equal to 3,500 calories. Add this number of calories to those you need to balance your energy requirements and you will gain one pound; subtract it and you will lose a pound.

Other Nutrients

Carbohydrates—which include sugars, starches, and acids—are only one of several chemical compounds in foods that yield calories. Proteins, found mainly in beef, poultry, and fish; fats, found in oils, butter, marbling of meat, poultry skin; and alcohol, found in some beverages, also contribute calories. Except for alcohol, most foods contain at least some of these nutrients.

The amount of carbohydrates varies from zero in meats and a trace in alcohol to a heavy concentration in sugar, syrups, some fruits, grains, and root vegetables.

As of this date, the most respected nutritional researchers insist that some carbohydrate is necessary every day for maintaining good health. The amount to be included is an individual matter, and in any drastic effort to change your eating patterns, be sure to consult your doctor first.

Now, on how to use this new language.

To begin with, you use this book like a dictionary. If your plan is to cut down on calories, the easiest way to do so is to consult the portable calorie counter and keep an accurate count of your total intake of food and beverages for a period of seven days. If you have not gained or lost weight during that week, divide that number by seven and you'll have your maintenance diet expressed in calories. To lose weight, you must reduce your daily or weekly intake of calories below this maintenance level. (To gain, increase the intake.)

Keeping in mind that you want to stay healthy and eat well-balanced meals (which include the basic food groups: milk or milk products; meat, poultry, or fish; vegetables and fruits; and whole grain or enriched breads or cereals, as well as some fats or oils), you then start to cut down on your portion in order to reduce your intake of calories. There are many imaginative ways to diet without total withdrawal from one's favorite foods.

Once you know and don't have to guess what calories are in your foods, you can relax and enjoy them. It could turn out that dieting isn't so bad after all.

ABBREVIATIONS AND SYMBOLS

---

* = prepared as package directs[1]
< = less than
& = and
" = inch
canned = bottles or jars as well as cans
dia. = diameter
fl. = fluid
liq. = liquid
lb. = pound
med. = medium

oz. = ounce
pkg. = package
pt. = pint
qt. = quart
sq. = square
T. = tablespoon
Tr. = trace
tsp. = teaspoon
wt. = weight

Italics or name in parentheses = registered trademark, ®. All data not identified by company or trademark are based on material obtained from the United States Department of Agriculture or Health, Education and Welfare/Food and Agriculture Organization.

EQUIVALENTS

By Weight	*By Volume*
1 pound = 16 ounces	1 quart = 4 cups
1 ounce = 28.35 grams	1 cup = 8 fluid ounces
3.52 ounces = 100 grams	1 cup = ½ pint
	1 cup = 16 tablespoons
	2 tablespoons = 1 fluid ounce
	1 tablespoon = 3 teaspoons
	1 pound butter = 4 sticks or 2 cups

---

[1]If the package directions call for whole or skim milk, the data given here are for whole milk unless otherwise stated.

A

Food and Description	Measure or Quantity	Calories
ABALONE, canned	4 oz.	91
AC'CENT	¼ tsp.	3
ALBACORE, raw, meat only	4 oz.	201
ALLSPICE (French's)	1 tsp.	6
ALMOND:		
In shell	10 nuts	60
Shelled, raw, natural, with skins	1 oz.	170
Roasted, dry (Planters)	1 oz.	170
Roasted, oil (Fisher)	1 oz.	178
ALMOND EXTRACT (Durkee) pure	1 tsp.	13
ALPHA-BITS, cereal (Post)	1 cup (1 oz.)	113
AMARETTO DI SARONNO	1 fl. oz.	82
ANCHOVY, PICKLED, canned, flat or rolled, not heavily salted, drained	2-oz. can	79
ANISE EXTRACT (Durkee) imitation	1 tsp.	16
ANISETTE:		
(DeKuyper)	1 fl. oz.	95
(Mr. Boston)	1 fl. oz.	88
APPLE:		
Eaten with skin	2½″ dia.	61
Eaten without skin	2½″ dia.	53
Canned (Comstock):		
Rings, drained	1 ring	30
Sliced	⅙ of 21-oz. can	45
Dried:		
(Del Monte)	1 cup	140
(Sun-Maid/Sunsweet)	2-oz. serving	150
Frozen, sweetened	1 cup	325
APPLE BROWN BETTY	1 cup	325
APPLE BUTTER (Smucker's) cider	1 T.	38
APPLE CIDER:		
Canned (Mott's) sweet	½ cup	59
Mix, Country Time	8 fl. oz.	98
APPLE-CRANBERRY DRINK (Hi-C):		
Canned	6 fl. oz.	90
*Mix	6 fl. oz.	72
APPLE-CRANBERRY JUICE, canned (Lincoln)	6 fl. oz.	100
APPLE DRINK:		
Canned:		

Food and Description	Measure or Quantity	Calories
Capri Sun, natural	6¾ fl. oz.	90
(Hi-C)	6 fl. oz.	92
*Mix (Hi-C)	6 fl. oz.	72
APPLE DUMPLINGS, Frozen		
(Pepperidge Farm)	1 dumpling	260
APPLE, ESCALLOPED, frozen		
(Stouffer's)	4 oz.	140
APPLE-GRAPE JUICE, canned:		
Musselman's	6 fl. oz.	82
(Red Cheek)	6 fl. oz.	69
APPLE JACKS, cereal (Kellogg's)	1 cup (1 oz.)	110
APPLE JAM (Smucker's)	1 T.	53
APPLE JELLY:		
Sweetened (Smucker's)	1 T.	67
Dietetic:		
(Dia-Mel; Featherweight;		
Louis Sherry)	1 T.	6
(Diet Delight)	1 T.	12
APPLE JUICE:		
Canned:		
(Lincoln)	6 fl. oz.	96
Musselman's	6 fl. oz.	80
(Ocean Spray)	6 fl. oz.	90
(Red Cheek)	6 fl. oz.	83
Chilled (Minute Maid)	6 fl. oz.	100
*Frozen:		
(Minute Maid)	6 fl. oz.	100
(Seneca Foods) Vitamin C added	6 fl. oz.	90
APPLE PIE (See Pie, Apple)		
APPLE SAUCE:		
Regular:		
(Del Monte)	½ cup	90
(Mott's):		
Natural style	½ cup	115
With ground cranberries	½ cup	110
Musselman's	½ cup	96
Dietetic:		
(Del Monte, Lite; Diet Delight)	½ cup	50
(S&W) *Nutradiet*, white		
or blue label	½ cup	55
APPLE STRUDEL, frozen		
(Pepperidge Farm)	3 oz.	240
APRICOT:		
Fresh, whole	1 apricot	18
Canned, regular pack:		
(Del Monte) whole, or halves,		
peeled	½ cup	200
(Stokely-Van Camp)	1 cup	220

2

Food and Description	Measure or Quantity	Calories
Canned, dietetic, solids & liq.:		
(Del Monte) Lite	½ cup	64
(Diet Delight):		
Juice pack	½ cup	60
Water pack	½ cup	35
(Featherweight):		
Juice pack	½ cup	50
Water pack	½ cup	35
(Libby's) Lite	½ cup	60
(S & W) Nutradiet:		
Halves, white or blue label	½ cup	50
Whole, juice	½ cup	40
Dried:		
(Del Monte; Sun-Maid; Sunsweet)	2 oz.	140
APRICOT LIQUEUR (DeKuyper)	1 fl. oz.	82
APRICOT NECTAR:		
(Del Monte)	6 fl. oz.	100
(Libby's)	6 fl. oz.	110
APRICOT-PINEAPPLE NECTAR, canned, dietetic (S&W) Nutradiet, blue label	6 oz.	35
APRICOT & PINEAPPLE PRESERVE OR JAM:		
Sweetened (Smucker's)	1 T.	53
Dietetic:		
(Diet Delight; Louis Sherry)	1 T.	6
(S&W) Nutradiet	1 T.	12
ARBY'S:		
Bac'n Cheddar Deluxe	1 sandwich	560
Beef & Cheddar Sandwich	6 oz.	450
Chicken breast sandwich	7¼-oz. sandwich	584
French Dip	5½-oz. sandwich	386
French fries	1½-oz. serving	216
Ham 'N Cheese	1 sandwich	380
Potato cakes	2 pieces	190
Roast Beef:		
Regular	5 oz.	350
Junior	3 oz.	220
Super	9¼ oz.	620
Sauce:		
Arby's	1 oz.	30
Horsey	1 oz.	100
ARTICHOKE:		
Boiled	15-oz. artichoke	187
Canned (Cara Mia) marinated, drained	6-oz. jar	175
Frozen (Birds Eye) deluxe	⅓ pkg.	39
ASPARAGUS:		

Food and Description	Measure or Quantity	Calories
Boiled	1 spear (½" dia. at base)	3
Canned, regular pack, solid & liq.:		
(Del Monte) spears, green or white	½ cup	20
(Green Giant)	8-oz. can	46
Canned, dietetic, solids & liq.:		
(Diet Delight)	½ cup	16
(Featherweight) cut spears	1 cup	40
(S&W) *Nutradiet*	1 cup	40
Frozen:		
(Birds Eye):		
Cuts	⅓ pkg.	29
Spears, regular or jumbo deluxe	⅓ pkg.	30
(Green Giant) cuts, butter sauce	3 oz.	57
(McKenzie)	⅓ pkg.	25
(Stouffer's) souffle	⅓ pkg.	115
AUNT JEMIMA SYRUP (See Syrup)		
AVOCADO, all varieties	1 fruit (10.7 oz.)	378
AWAKE (Birds Eye)	6 fl. oz.	84
AYDS:		
Butterscotch	1 piece	27
Chocolate, chocolate mint, vanilla	1 piece	26

B

Food and Description	Measure or Quantity	Calories
BACON, broiled:		
(Hormel) *Black Label*	1 slice	30
(Oscar Mayer):		
Regular slice	6-gram slice	35
Thick slice	1 slice	64
BACON BITS:		
Bac*Os (Betty Crocker)	1 tsp.	13
(French's) imitation	1 tsp.	6
(Hormel)	1 tsp.	10
(Libby's) crumbles	1 tsp.	8
(Oscar Mayer) real	1 tsp.	6
BACON, CANADIAN, unheated:		
(Eckrich)	1 oz.	35
(Hormel) sliced	1 oz.	45
(Oscar Mayer) 93% fat free:		
Thin	.7-oz. slice	30
Thick	1-oz. slice	40
BACON, SIMULATED, cooked:		
(Oscar Mayer) *Lean'N Tasty:*		
Beef	1 slice	39
Pork	1 slice	45
(Swift's) *Sizzlean*	1 strip	50
BAGEL:		
Egg	3-inch dia., 1.9 oz.	162
Water	3-inch dia., 1.9 oz.	163
BAKING POWDER:		
(Calumet)	1 tsp.	2
(Featherweight) low sodium, cereal free	1 tsp.	8
BAMBOO SHOOTS:		
Raw, trimmed	4 oz.	31
Canned, drained (La Choy)	½ cup	6
BANANA, medium (Dole)	6.3-oz. banana (weighed unpeeled)	101
BANANA EXTRACT (Durkee) imitation	1 tsp.	15
BANANA NECTAR (Libby's)	6 fl. oz.	60
BANANA PIE (See PIE, Banana)		
BARBECUE SEASONING (French's)	1 tsp.	6

5

Food and Description	Measure or Quantity	Calories
BARBERA WINE (Louis M. Martini) 12½% alcohol	3 fl. oz.	66
BARLEY, pearled (Quaker Scotch)	¼ cup	172
BASIL (French's)	1 tsp.	3
BASS:		
Baked, stuffed	3½″ × 4½″ × 1½″	531
Oven-fried	8¾″ × 4½″ × ⅝″	392
BAY LEAF (French's)	1 tsp.	5
B & B LIQUEUR	1 fl. oz.	94
B.B.Q. SAUCE & BEEF, frozen (Banquet) *Cookin' Bag*, sliced	4-oz. serving	133
BEAN, BAKED:		
(USDA):		
With pork & molasses sauce	1 cup	382
With pork & tomato sauce	1 cup	311
Canned:		
(B&M):		
Pea bean with pork in brown sugar sauce	8 oz.	345
Red kidney bean in brown sugar sauce	8 oz.	325
(Campbell):		
Home style	8-oz. can	270
With pork & tomato sauce	8-oz. can	270
(Friend's)		
Pea	9-oz. serving	363
Yellow eye	9-oz. serving	353
(Grandma Brown's)	8 oz.	289
(Howard Johnson's)	1 cup	340
BEAN, BARBECUE (Campbell)	7⅞-oz. can	678
BEAN, BLACK OR BROWN, dry	1 cup	678
BEAN & FRANKFURTER, canned:		
(Campbell) in tomato and molasses sauce	7⅞-oz. can	350
(Hormel) *Short Orders*, 'n wieners	7½-oz. can	280
BEAN & FRANKFURTER DINNER, frozen:		
(Banquet)	10¼-oz. dinner	500
(Swanson) *TV Brand*	11¼-oz. dinner	490
BEAN, GARBANZO, canned, dietetic (S&W) *Nutradiet,* low sodium, green label	½ cup	105
BEAN, GREEN:		
boiled, 1½″ to 2″ pieces, drained	½ cup	17
Canned, regular pack, solids & liq.:		
(Del Monte)	4 oz.	20
(Green Giant) French or whole	½ cup	21

6

Food and Description	Measure or Quantity	Calories
(Libby's) French	½ cup	21
(Sunshine)	½ cup	20
Canned, dietetic, solids & liq.:		
(Del Monte) No Salt Added	4 oz.	19
(Diet Delight; S&W, *Nutradiet*)	½ cup	20
Frozen:		
(Birds Eye):		
Cut or French	⅓ pkg.	30
French, with almonds	⅓ pkg.	34
Whole, deluxe	⅓ pkg.	26
(Green Giant):		
Cut or French, with butter sauce	½ cup	40
Cut, *Harvest Fresh*	½ cup	25
With mushroom in cream sauce	½ cup	80
(Seabrook Farms; Southland)	⅓ pkg.	29
BEAN, GREEN & MUSHROOM CASSEROLE (Stouffer's)	½ pkg.	150
BEAN, GREEN, WITH POTATOES, canned (Sunshine) solids & liq.	½ cup	34
BEAN, ITALIAN:		
Canned (Del Monte) solids & liq.	4 oz.	25
Frozen (Birds Eye)	⅓ pkg.	38
BEAN, KIDNEY:		
Canned, regular pack, solids & liq.		
(Furman) red, fancy, light	½ cup	121
(Van Camp):		
Light	8 oz.	194
New Orleans style	8 oz.	188
Red	8 oz.	213
Canned, dietetic (S&W) *Nutradiet*, low sodium,	½ cup	90
BEAN, LIMA:		
Boiled, drained	½ cup	94
Canned, regular pack, solids & liq.:		
(Del Monte)	4 oz.	70
(Libby's)	½ cup	91
(Sultana) butter bean	¼ of 15-oz. can	82
Canned, dietetic (Featherweight)	½ cup	80
Frozen:		
(Birds Eye) baby	⅓ pkg.	130
(Green Giant):		
In butter sauce	½ cup	120
Harvest Fresh or polybag	½ cup	100
(Seabrook Farms):		
Baby lima	⅓ pkg.	126

7

Food and Description	Measure or Quantity	Calories
Baby butter bean	⅓ pkg.	139
Fordhooks	⅓ pkg.	98
BEAN, REFRIED, canned:		
Old El Paso:		
Plain	4 oz.	106
With sausage	4 oz.	224
(Ortega) lightly spicy or true bean	½ cup	170
BEAN SALAD, canned		
(Green Giant)	¼-oz. serving	80
BEAN SOUP (See SOUP, Bean)		
BEAN SPROUT:		
Mung, raw	½ lb.	80
Mung, boiled, drained	¼ lb.	32
Soy, raw	½ lb.	104
Soy, boiled, drained	¼ lb.	43
Canned (La Choy)	⅔ cup	8
BEAN, YELLOW OR WAX:		
Boiled, 1″ pieces, drained	½ cup	18
Canned, regular pack, solids & liq.:		
(Comstock)	½ cup	22
(Del Monte) cut or french	½ cup	18
(Libby's) cut	4 oz.	23
(Stokley-Van Camp)	½ cup	23
Canned, dietetic (Featherweight)		
cut, solids & liq.	½ cup	25
BEEF, choice grade, medium done:		
Brisket, braised:		
Lean & fat	3 oz.	350
Lean only	3 oz.	189
Chuck, pot roast:		
Lean & fat	3 oz.	278
Lean only	3 oz.	182
Fat, separable, cooked	1 oz.	207
Filet Mignon (See Steak, sirloin, lean)		
Flank, braised, 100% lean	3 oz.	167
Ground:		
Regular, raw	½ cup	303
Regular, broiled	3 oz.	243
Lean, broiled	3 oz.	186
Rib:		
Roasted, lean & fat	3 oz.	374
Lean only	3 oz.	205
Round:		
Broiled, lean & fat	3 oz.	222
Lean only	3 oz.	161
Rump:		
Broiled, lean & fat	3 oz.	295
Lean only	3 oz.	177

Food and Description	Measure or Quantity	Calories
Steak, club, broiled:		
One 8-oz. steak (weighed without bone before cooking) will give you:		
Lean & fat	5.9 oz.	754
Lean only	3.4 oz.	234
Steak, porterhouse, broiled:		
One 16-oz. steak (weighed with bone before cooking) will give you:		
Lean & fat	10.2 oz.	1339
Lean only	5.9 oz.	372
Steak, ribeye, broiled:		
One 10-oz. steak (weighed without bone before cooking) will give you:		
Lean & fat	7.3 oz.	911
Lean only	3.8 oz.	258
Steak, sirloin, double-bone, broiled:		
One 16-oz. steak (weighed with bone before cooking will give you:		
Lean & fat	8.9 oz.	1028
Lean only	5.9 oz.	359
One 12-oz. steak (weighed with bone before cooking) will give you:		
Lean & fat	6.6 oz.	767
Lean only	4.4 oz.	268
Steak, T-bone, broiled:		
One 16-oz. steak (weighed with bone before cooking) will give you:		
Lean & fat	9.8 oz.	1315
Lean only	5.5 oz.	348
BEEF BOUILLON:		
(Herb-Ox):		
Cube	1 cube	6
Packet	1 packet	8
MBT	1 packet	14
Low sodium (Featherweight)	1 tsp.	18
BEEF, CHIPPED:		
Cooked, home recipe	½ cup	188
Frozen, creamed:		
(Banquet) *Cookin' Bag*	5-oz. pkg.	160
(Stouffer's)	5½-oz. serving	231
BEEF DINNER or ENTREE, frozen:		
(Banquet):		
American Favorites, chopped	11-oz. dinner	434

Food and Description	Measure or Quantity	Calories
Extra Helping, regular (Green Giant)	16-oz. dinner	864
Baked, boneless ribs in BBQ sauce with corn on the cob	1 meal	390
Twin pouch, burgundy, with rice & carrots	1 meal	280
(Morton):		
Regular	10-oz. dinner	260
Country Table, sliced	14-oz. dinner	510
(Stouffer's) Lean Cuisine, oriental	8⅝-oz. pkg.	280
(Swanson):		
Hungry Man, sliced	12¼-oz. entree	300
TV Brand, chopped sirloin	10-oz. dinner	380
3-course	15-oz. dinner	450
(Weight Watchers):		
Beefsteak, 2-compartment meal	9¾-oz. pkg.	320
Oriental	10-oz. meal	260
Sirloin in mushroom sauce, 3-compartment meal	13-oz. pkg.	410
BEEF, DRIED, canned:		
(Hormel)	1 oz.	45
(Swift)	1 oz.	47
BEEF GOULASH (Hormel) Short Orders	7½-oz. can	230
BEEF, GROUND, SEASONING MIX:		
*(Durkee):		
Regular	1 cup	653
With onion	1 cup	659
(French's) with onion	1⅛-oz. pkg.	100
BEEF HASH, ROAST:		
Canned, Mary Kitchen (Hormel):		
Regular	7½-oz. serving	350
Short Orders	7½-oz. can	360
Frozen (Stouffer's)	½ of 11½-oz. pkg.	265
BEEF PEPPER ORIENTAL, frozen (La Choy):		
Dinner	12-oz. dinner	250
Entree	12-oz. entree	160
BEEF PIE, frozen:		
(Banquet):		
Regular	8-oz. pie	557
Supreme	8-oz. pie	380
(Morton)	8-oz. pie	320
(Swanson):		
Regular	8-oz. pie	400
Hungry Man	16-oz. pie	720
BEEF PUFFS, frozen (Durkee)	1 piece	47

Food and Description	Measure or Quantity	Calories
BEEF ROLL (Hormel) Lumberjack	1 oz.	101
BEEF, SHORT RIBS, frozen (Stouffer's) boneless, with vegetable gravy	½ of 11½-oz. pkg.	350
BEEF SOUP (See SOUP, Beef)		
BEEF SPREAD, ROAST, canned (Underwood)	½ of 4¾-oz. can	140
BEEF STEAK, BREADED (Hormel) frozen	4-oz. serving	370
BEEF STEW:		
Home recipe, made with lean beef chuck	1 cup	218
Canned, regular pack:		
Dinty Moore (Hormel):		
Regular	8-oz. serving	210
Short Orders	7½-oz. can	150
(Libby's)	7½-oz serving	160
(Swanson)	7⅝-oz. serving	150
Canned, dietetic (Dia Mel)	8-oz. serving	200
Frozen:		
(Banquet) Buffet Supper	2-lb. pkg.	1016
(Green Giant:		
Boil'N Bag	9-oz. entree	180
Twin pouch, with noodles	9-oz. entree	333
(Stouffer's)	10-oz. serving	305
BEEF STEW SEASONING MIX:		
*(Durkee)	1 cup	379
(French's)	1 pkg.	150
BEEF STOCK BASE (French's)	1 tsp.	8
BEEF STIX (Vienna)	1 oz.	163
BEEF STROGANOFF, frozen (Stouffer's) with parlsey noodles	9¾ oz.	390
***BEEF STROGANOFF SEASONING MIX** (Durkee)	1 cup	820
BEER & ALE:		
Regular:		
Black Horse Ale	8 fl. oz.	108
Budweiser; Busch Bavarian	8 fl. oz.	100
Michelob	8 fl. oz.	113
Pearl Premium	8 fl. oz.	99
Stroh Bohemian	8 fl. oz.	84
Light or low carbohydrate:		
Budweiser Light; Natural light	8 fl. oz.	75
Gablinger's	8 fl. oz.	66
Michelob Light	8 fl. oz.	90
Pearl Light	8 fl. oz.	68
Stroh Light	8 fl. oz.	77
BEER, NEAR:		

11

Food and Description	Measure or Quantity	Calories
Goetz Pale	8 fl. oz.	53
Kingsbury (Heileman)	8 fl. oz.	30
(Metbrew)	8 fl. oz.	49
BEET:		
Boiled, whole	2" dia. beet	16
Boiled, sliced	½ cup	33
Canned, regular pack, solids & liq.:		
(Del Monte)		
Pickled	4 oz.	77
Sliced	4 oz.	29
(Greenwood)		
Harvard	½ cup	70
Pickled	½ cup	110
(Stokely-Van Camp) pickled	½ cup	95
Canned, dietetic, solids & liq.:		
(Blue Boy) whole	½ cup	39
(Comstock)	½ cup	30
(Featherweight) sliced	½ cup	45
(S&W) *Nutradiet*, sliced	½ cup	35
BENEDICTINE LIQUEUR (Julius Wile)	1½ fl. oz.	168
BIG H, burger sauce (Hellmann's)	1 T.	71
BIG MAC (See (*McDONALD'S*)		
BIG WHEEL (Hostess)	1 piece	170
BISCUIT DOUGH (Pillsbury):		
Baking Powder, *1869 Brand*	1 biscuit	100
Big Country	1 biscuit	95
Big Country, Good 'N Buttery	1 biscuit	100
Buttermilk:		
Regular	1 biscuit	50
Ballard, Oven Ready	1 biscuit	50
Extra Lights	1 biscuit	60
Extra rich, *Hungry Jack*	1 biscuit	65
Fluffy, *Hungry Jack*	1 biscuit	100
Butter Tastin', *1869 Brand*	1 biscuit	100
Dinner	1 biscuit	55
Flaky, *Hungry Jack*	1 biscuit	90
Oven Ready, Ballard	1 biscuit	50
BITTERS (Angostura)	1 tsp.	14
BLACKBERRY, fresh, hulled	1 cup	84
BLACKBERRY JELLY:		
Sweetened (Smucker's)	1 T.	53
Dietetic:		
(Diet Delight)	1 T.	12
(Featherweight)	1 T.	16
BLACKBERRY LIQUEUR (Bols)	1 fl. oz.	95
BLACKBERRY PRESERVE OR JAM:		

Food and Description	Measure or Quantity	Calories
Sweetened (Smucker's)	1 T.	53
Dietetic:		
(Dia-Mel; Louis Sherry)	1 T.	6
(Featherweight)	1 T.	16
(S&W) *Nutradiet*	1 T.	12
BLACKBERRY WINE (Mogen David)	3 fl. oz.	135
BLACK-EYED PEAS:		
Canned, with pork, solids & liq. (Sunshine)	½ cup	90
Frozen:		
(Birds Eye)	⅓ of pkg.	133
(McKenzie; Seabrook Farms)	⅓ pkg.	130
(Southland)	⅓ of 16-oz. pkg.	120
BLINTZE, frozen (King Kold) cheese	2½-oz. piece	132
BLOODY MARY MIX:		
Dry (Bar-Tender's)	1 serving	26
Liquid (Sacramento)	5½-fl. oz. can	39
BLUEBERRY, fresh, whole	½ cup	45
BLUEBERRY PIE (See PIE, Blueberry)		
BLUEBERRY PRESERVE OR JAM:		
Sweetened (Smucker's)	1 T.	53
Dietetic (Louis Sherry)	1 T.	6
BLUEFISH, broiled	3½″ × 3″ × ½″ piece	199
BODY BUDDIES, cereal (General Mills):		
Brown sugar & honey	1 cup	110
Natural fruit flavor	¾ cup	110
BOLOGNA:		
(Eckrich):		
Beef:		
Regular, garlic	1 oz.	90
Thick slice	1½-oz. slice	140
German brand	1-oz. slice	80
Meat, regular	1-oz. slice	90
(Hormel):		
Beef	1-oz. slice	85
Meat	1-oz. slice	90
(Oscar Mayer):		
Beef	8-oz. slice	73
Beef	1-oz. slice	90
Meat	1-oz. slice	91
(Swift)	1-oz. slice	95
BOLOGNA & CHEESE:		
(Eckrich)	.7-oz. slice	90
(Oscar Mayer)	.8-oz. slice	73

Food and Description	Measure or Quantity	Calories
BONITO, canned (Star-Kist):		
Chunk	6½-oz. can	605
Solid	7-oz. can	650
BOO*BERRY, cereal (General Mills)	1 cup	110
BORSCHT, canned:		
Regular:		
(Gold's)	8-oz. serving	72
(Mother's) old fashioned	8.oz. serving	90
Dietetic or low calorie:		
Gold's)	8-oz. serving	24
(Mother's):		
Artificially sweetened	8-oz. serving	29
Unsalted	8-oz. serving	107
(Rokeach)	8-oz. serving	27
BOSCO (See SYRUP)		
BOYSENBERRY JELLY:		
Sweetened (Smucker's)	1 T.	53
Dietetic (S&W) *Nutradiet,* red label	1 T.	12
BRAN:		
Crude	1 oz.	60
Miller's (Elam's)	1 oz.	87
BRAN BREAKFAST CEREAL:		
(Kellogg's):		
All Bran or *Bran Buds*	⅓ cup	70
Cracklin' Oat Bran	½ cup	120
40% bran flakes	¾ cup	90
Raisin	¾ cup	110
(Nabisco)	½ cup	70
(Post) 40% bran flakes	⅔ cup	107
(Quaker) *Corn Bran*	⅔ cup	109
(Ralston-Purina):		
Bran Chex	⅔ cup	90
40% bran	¾ cup	100
Raisin	¾ cup	120
BRANDY, FLAVORED		
(Mr. Boston):		
Apricot	1 fl. oz.	94
Blackberry	1 fl. oz.	92
Cherry	1 fl. oz.	87
Ginger	1 fl. oz.	72
Peach	1 fl. oz.	94
BRAUNSCHWEIGER:		
(Eckrich) chub	1 oz.	70
(Oscar Mayer) chub	1 oz.	98
(Swfit) 8-oz. chub	1 oz.	109
BRAZIL NUT:		
Shelled	4 nuts	114

Food and Description	Measure or Quantity	Calories
Roasted (Fisher) salted	1 oz.	193
BREAD:		
Apple (Pepperidge Farm) with cinnamon	.9-oz. slice	70
Boston Brown	3″ × ¾″ slice	101
Bran (Pepperidge Farm) with raisins	.9-oz. slice	65
Cinnamon (Pepperidge Farm)	.9-oz. slice	80
Corn & Molasses (Pepperidge Farm)	.9-oz. slice	75
Cracked wheat:		
(Pepperidge Farm)	.9-oz. slice	75
(Wonder)	1-oz. slice	70
Crispbread, *Wasa:*		
Mora	3.2-oz. slice	333
Rye, lite	.3-oz. slice	30
Sesame	.5-oz. slice	50
Date-nut roll (Dromedary)	1-oz. slice	80
Date walnut (Pepperidge Farm)	.9-oz. slice	75
Flatbread, *Ideal:*		
Bran	.2-oz. slice	19
Extra thin	.1-oz. slice	12
Whole grain	.2-oz. slice	19
French:		
(Pepperidge Farm) fully baked	2-oz. slice	150
(Wonder)	1-oz. slice	70
Hillbilly	1-oz. slice	70
Hollywood, dark	1-oz. slice	70
Honey bran (Pepperidge Farm)	1 slice	95
Honey wheat berry (Arnold)	1.2-oz. slice	90
Italian (Pepperidge Farm) brown & serve	1.3-oz. slice	110
Oat (Arnold) *Bran'nola*	1.3-oz. slice	110
Oatmeal (Pepperidge Farm)	.9-oz. slice	70
Orange & Raisin (Pepperidge Farm)	.9-oz. slice	70
Protein (*Thomas'*)	.7-oz. slice	46
Pumpernickel:		
(Arnold)	1-oz. slice	75
(Levy's)	1.1-oz. slice	85
(Pepperidge Farm):		
Regular	1.1-oz. slice	85
Party	.2-oz. slice	17
Raisin:		
(Arnold) tea	.9-oz. slice	70
(Pepperidge Farm)	1 slice	75
(Sun-Maid)	1-oz. slice	80
(Thomas') cinnamon	.8-oz. slice	60
Roman Meal	1-oz. slice	70

Food and Description	Measure or Quantity	Calories
Rye:		
(Arnold) Jewish	1.1-oz. slice	75
(Levy's) Real	1-oz. slice	80
(Pepperidge Farm) family	1.1-oz. slice	85
(Wonder)	1-oz. slice	70
Sahara (Thomas') wheat or white	1-oz. piece	85
Sourdough, *Di Carlo*	1-oz. slice	70
Sprouted wheat (Pepperidge Farm)	.9-oz. slice	113
Vienna (Pepperidge Farm)	.9-oz. slice	175
Wheat (see also Cracked Wheat or Whole Wheat):		
(Arnold) *Bran'nola*	1.3-oz. slice	105
Fresh Horizons	1-oz. slice	50
Fresh & Natural	1-oz. slice	70
Home Pride	1-oz. slice	70
(Pepperidge Farm) sandwich	.8-oz. slice	55
(Wonder) family	1-oz. slice	70
Wheatberry, *Home Pride,* honey	1-oz. slice	70
Wheat Germ (Pepperidge Farm)	.9-oz. slice	70
White:		
(Arnold):		
Brick Oven	.8-oz. slice	65
Measure Up	.5-oz. slice	40
Home Pride	1-oz. slice	72
(Pepperidge Farm):		
Large loaf	.9-oz. slice	75
Sandwich	.8-oz. slice	65
Sliced, 1-lb. loaf	.9-oz. slice	75
Toasting	1.2-oz. slice	85
(Wonder) regular	1-oz. slice	70
Whole wheat:		
(Arnold) *Brick Oven*	.8-oz. slice	60
(Pepperidge Farm) thin slice	1 slice	70
(Thomas') 100%	.8-oz. slice	56
BREAD, CANNED, brown, plain or raisin (B&M)	½" slice	80
BREAD CRUMBS:		
(Contadina) seasoned	½ cup	211
(Pepperidge Farm)	1 oz.	110
***BREAD DOUGH:**		
Frozen:		
(Pepperidge Farm):		
Country rye or white	1/10 of loaf	80
Stone ground wheat	1/10 of loaf	75
(Rich's):		
French	1/20 of loaf	59
Italian	1/20 of loaf	60
Refrigerated (Pillsbury):		
Poppin' Fresh	1/16 of loaf	110

Food and Description	Measure or Quantity	Calories
*BREAD MIX (Pillsbury):		
Applesauce spice, banana or blueberry nut	¹⁄₁₂ of loaf	150
Cherry nut or nut	¹⁄₁₂ of loaf	170
Cranberry or date	¹⁄₁₂ of loaf	160
BREAD PUDDING, with raisins	½ cup	248
*BREAD STICK DOUGH (Pillsbury)		
Pipin' Hot	1 piece	100
BREAKFAST BAR (Carnation):		
Almond crunch	1 piece	210
All other varieties	1 piece	200
*BREAKFAST DRINK (Pillsbury)	1 pouch	290
BREAKFAST SQUARES (General Mills) all flavors	1 bar	190
BROCCOLI:		
Boiled, while stalk	1 stalk (6.3 oz.)	47
Boiled, ½" pieces	½ cup	20
Frozen:		
(Birds Eye):		
In cheese sauce	⅓ pkg.	87
Chopped, cuts or florets	⅓ of pkg.	31
Spears in butter sauce	⅓ of pkg.	58
(Green Giant):		
Cuts, polybag	½ cup	18
Spears in butter sauce	3⅓ oz.	40
Spears, mini, *Harvest Fresh*	⅛ of pkg.	16
Frozen:		
(Seabrook Farms) chopped or spears	⅓ pkg.	30
(Stouffer's) in cheese sauce	½ of 9-oz. pkg.	130
BROTH & SEASONING:		
(George Washington)	1 packet	5
Maggi	1 T.	22
BRUSSELS SPROUT:		
Boiled	3-4 sprouts	28
Frozen:		
(Birds Eye):		
Regular	⅓ of pkg.	6
Baby, with cheese sauce	⅓ pkg.	104
Baby, deluxe	⅓ pkg.	49
(Green Giant):		
In butter sauce	½ cup	60
Halves in cheese sauce	½ cup	80
BUCKWHEAT, cracked (Pocono)	1 oz.	104
BUC*WHEATS, cereal (General Mills)	1 oz. (¾ cup)	110
BULGUR, canned, seasoned	4 oz.	206

Food and Description	Measure or Quantity	Calories
BURGER KING:		
Apple pie	3-oz. pie	240
Cheeseburger	1 burger	350
Cheeseburger, double meat	1 burger	530
Coca-Cola	1 medium-sized drink	121
French fries	1 regular order	210
Hamburger	1 burger	290
Onion rings	1 regular order	270
Pepsi, diet	1 medium-sized drink	7
Shake, chocolate or vanilla	1 shake	340
Whopper:		
Regular	1 burger	630
Regular, with cheese	1 burger	740
Double Beef	1 burger	850
Double beef, with cheese	1 burger	950
Junior	1 burger	370
Junior with cheese	1 burger	420
BURGUNDY WINE:		
(Louis M. Martini)	3 fl. oz.	60
(Paul Masson)	3 fl. oz.	70
(Taylor)	3 fl. oz.	75
BURGUNDY WINE, SPARKLING:		
(B&G)	3 fl. oz.	69
(Great Western)	3 fl. oz.	82
(Taylor)	3 fl. oz.	78
BURRITO:		
*Canned (Del Monte)	1 burrito	310
Frozen:		
(Hormel):		
Beef	1 burrito	220
Cheese	1 burrito	250
Hot chili	1 burrito	210
(Van de Kamp's) regular & guacamole sauce	6-oz. serving	350
BURRITO FILLING MIX, canned		
(Del Monte)	½ cup	110
BUTTER:		
Regular:		
(Breakstone)	1 T.	100
(Meadow Gold)	1 tsp.	35
Whipped (Breakstone)	1 T.	67
BUTTERSCOTCH MORSELS		
(Nestlé)	1 oz.	150

C

Food and Description	Measure or Quantity	Calories
CABBAGE:		
Boiled, until tender, without salt, drained	1 cup	29
Canned, solids & liq.:		
(Comstock) red	½ cup	60
(Greenwood)	½ cup	60
Frozen (Green Giant) stuffed	½ of pkg.	220
CABERNET SAUVIGNON:		
(Louis M. Martini)	3 fl. oz.	63
(Paul Masson)	3 fl. oz.	70
CAFE COMFORT, 55 proof	1 fl. oz.	79
CAKE:		
Regular, non-frozen:		
Plain, home recipe, with butter, with boiled white icing	⅑ of 9″ square	401
Angel food, home recipe	1/12 of 8″ cake	108
Caramel, home recipe, with caramel icing	⅑ of 9″ square	322
Chocolate, home recipe, with chocolate icing, 2-layer	1/12 of 9″ cake	365
Crumb (Hostess)	1¼-oz. cake	130
Fruit:		
Home recipe, dark	1/30 of 8″ loaf	57
Home recipe, made with butter	1/30 of 8″ loaf	58
(Holland Honey Cake) unsalted	1/14 of cake	80
Pound, home recipe, traditional, made with butter	3½″ × 3½″ slice	123
Raisin Date Loaf (Holland Honey Cake) low sodium	1/14 of 13-oz. cake	8
Sponge, home recipe	1/12 of 10″ cake	196
White, home recipe, made with butter, without icing, 2-layer	⅑ of 9″ wide, 3″ wide cake	353
Yellow, home recipe, made with butter, without icing, 2-layer	1/19 of cake	351
Frozen:		
Apple Walnut:		
(Pepperidge Farm) with cream cheese icing	⅛ of 11¾ oz. cake	150

19

Food and Description	Measure or Quantity	Calories
(Sara Lee)	⅛ of 12½-oz. cake	165
Banana (Sara Lee)	⅛ of 13¾-oz. cake	175
Carrot:		
(Pepperidge Farm)	⅛ of 11¾-oz. cake	140
(Weight Watchers)	2⅝-oz. serving	153
Cheesecake:		
(Morton) *Great Little Desserts:*		
Cherry	6 oz.-cake	460
Cream cheese	6-oz. cake	480
Strawberry	6-oz. cake	470
(Rich's) Viennese	1/14 of 42-oz. cake	230
(Sara Lee):		
Blueberry, *For 2*	½ of 11.3-oz. cake	425
Cream cheese:		
Regular	⅓ of 10-oz. cake	281
Cherry	⅙ of 19-oz. cake	225
Strawberry	⅙ of 19-oz. cake	223
Strawberry, *For 2*	½ of 11.3-oz. cake	420
(Weight Watchers):		
Regular	4-oz. serving	172
Strawberry	4-oz. serving	153
Chocolate:		
(Pepperidge Farm):		
Layer, fudge	1/10 of 17-oz. cake	190
Supreme	¼ of 11½-oz. cake	310
(Sara Lee):		
Regular	⅛ of 13¼-oz. cake	199
German	⅛ of 12¼-oz. cake	173
Coconut (Pepperidge Farm) layer	1/10 of 17-oz. cake	180
Coffee (Sara Lee):		
Almond	⅛ of 11¾-oz. cake	165
Almond ring	⅛ of 9½-oz. cake	135
Apple	⅛ of 15-oz. cake	175
Butter, *For 2*	½ of 6½-oz. cake	356
Pecan	⅛ of 11¼-oz. cake	173
Streusel, butter	⅛ of 11½-oz. cake	164
Crumb (See ROLL OR BUN, Crumb)		
Devil's food (Pepperidge Farm) layer	1/10 of 17-oz. cake	180
Golden (Pepperidge Farm) layer	1/10 of 17-oz. cake	180
Lemon coconut (Pepperidge Farm)	¼ of 12¼-oz. cake	280
Orange (Sara See)	⅛ of 13¾-oz. cake	179
Pound:		
(Pepperidge Farm) butter	1/10 of 10¾-oz. cake	130

Food and Description	Measure or Quantity	Calories
(Sara Lee):		
Regular	1/10 of 10¾-oz. cake	125
Banana nut	1/10 of 11-oz. cake	117
Chocolate	1/10 of 10¾-oz. cake	122
Family size	1/15 of 16½-oz. cake	127
Homestyle	1/10 of 9½-oz. cake	114
Spice (Weight Watchers)	2⅝-oz. serving	157
Strawberry cream (Pepperidge Farm) Supreme	1/12 of 12-oz. cake	190
Strawberries'n cream, layer (Sara Lee)	1/8 of 20½-oz. cake	218
Torte (Sara Lee):		
Apples'n cream	1/8 of 21-oz. cake	203
Fudge & nut	1/8 of 15¾-oz. cake	200
Vanilla (Pepperidge Farm) layer	1/10 of 17-oz. cake	180
Walnut, layer (Sara Lee)	1/8 of 18-oz. cake	210
CAKE OR COOKIE ICING		
(Pillsbury) all flavors	1 T.	70
CAKE ICING:		
Butter pecan (Betty Crocker) *Creamy Deluxe*	1/12 of can	170
Caramel, home recipe	4 oz.	408
Cherry (Betty Crocker) *Creamy Deluxe*	1/12 of can	170
Chocolate:		
(Betty Crocker) *Creamy Deluxe:*		
Regular, chip or milk	1/12 of can	170
Sour cream	1/12 of can	160
(Duncan Hines) regular or milk	1/12 of can	163
(Pillsbury) *Frosting Supreme,* fudge, nut or milk	1/12 of can	150
Coconut almond (Pillsbury) *Frosting Supreme*	1/12 of can	150
Cream cheese:		
(Betty Crocker) *Creamy Deluxe*	1/12 of can	170
(Pillsbury) *Frosting Supreme*	1/12 of can	160
Double dutch (Pillsbury) *Frosting Supreme*	1/12 of can	150
Orange (Betty Crocker) *Creamy Deluxe*	1/12 of can	170
Strawberry (Pillsbury) *Frosting Supreme*	1/12 of can	160
Vanilla:		
(Betty Crocker) *Creamy Deluxe*	1/12 of can	170
(Duncan Hines)	1/12 of can	163
(Pillsbury) *Frosting Supreme,* regular or sour cream	1/12 of can	160

21

Food and Description	Measure or Quantity	Calories
White:		
Home recipe, boiled	4 oz.	358
Home recipe, uncooked	4 oz.	426
(Betty Crocker) *Creamy Deluxe*	¹⁄₁₂ of can	160
CAKE ICING MIX:		
Regular:		
Banana (Betty Crocker) *Chiquita*, creamy	¹⁄₁₂ of pkg.	170
Butter Brickle (Betty Crocker) creamy	¹⁄₁₂ of pkg.	170
Butter pecan (Betty Crocker) creamy	¹⁄₁₂ of pkg.	170
Caramel (Pillsbury) *Rich'n Easy*	¹⁄₁₂ of pkg.	140
Cherry (Betty Crocker) creamy	¹⁄₁₂ of pkg.	170
Chocolate:		
Home recipe, fudge	½ cup	586
(Betty Crocker) Creamy:		
Fluffy, almond fudge	¹⁄₁₂ of pkg.	180
Fudge, creamy, dark or milk	¹⁄₁₂ of pkg.	170
(Pillsbury) *Rich'n Easy,* fudge or milk	¹⁄₁₂ of pkg.	160
Coconut almond (Pillsbury)	¹⁄₁₂ of pk.	160
Coconut pecan:		
(Betty Crocker) creamy	¹⁄₁₂ of pkg.	140
(Pillsbury)	¹⁄₁₂ of pkg.	150
Cream cheese & nut		
(Betty Crocker) creamy	¹⁄₁₂ of pkg.	150
Lemon:		
(Betty Crocker) *Sunkist,* creamy	¹⁄₁₂ of pkg.	170
(Pillsbury) *Rich'n Easy*	¹⁄₁₂ of pkg.	140
Strawberry (Pillsbury) *Rich'n Easy*	¹⁄₁₂ of pkg.	140
Vanilla (Pillsbury) *Rich'n Easy*	¹⁄₁₂ of pkg.	150
White:		
(Betty Crocker) fluffy	¹⁄₁₂ of pkg.	60
(Betty Crocker) sour cream, creamy	¹⁄₁₂ of pkg.	180
(Pillsbury) fluffy	¹⁄₁₂ of pkg.	60
CAKE MIX:		
Regular:		
*Apple (Pillsbury) *Streusel Swirl*	¹⁄₁₆ of cake	260
Angel Food:		
(Betty Crocker):		
Chocolate or one-step	¹⁄₁₂ pkg.	140
Traditional	¹⁄₁₂ pkg.	130
(Duncan Hines)	¹⁄₁₂ pkg.	124
*(Pillsbury) raspberry or white	¹⁄₁₂ of cake	140
Applesauce raisin (Betty Crocker) *Snackin' Cake*	⅑ pkg.	180

Food and Description	Measure or Quantity	Calories
*Applesauce spice (Pillsbury)	1/12 of cake	250
*Banana:		
(Betty Crocker) *Supermoist*	1/12 of cake	260
(Pillsbury) *Pillsbury Plus*	1/12 of cake	250
*Banana walnut (Betty Crocker)		
Snackin' Cake	1/9 of cake	90
*Boston cream (Pillsbury) *Bundt*	1/16 of cake	270
*Butter (Pillsbury):		
Pillsbury Plus	1/12 of cake	240
Streusel Swirl, rich	1/16 of cake	260
*Butter Brickle (Betty Crocker)		
Supermoist	1/12 of cake	260
*Butter pecan (Betty Crocker)		
Supermoist	1/12 of cake	250
*Carrot (Betty Crocker)		
Supermoist	1/12 of cake	260
*Carrot'n spice (Pillsbury)		
Pillsbury Plus	1/12 of cake	260
*Cheesecake (Jell-O)	1/8 of 8" cake	283
*Cherry chip (Betty Crocker)		
Supermoist	1/12 of cake	180
Chocolate:		
(Betty Crocker):		
*Pudding	1/6 of cake	230
Snackin' Cake:		
Almond	1/9 of pkg.	200
Fudge Chip	1/9 pkg.	190
Stir 'N Frost:		
With chocolate frosting	1/6 pkg.	220
Fudge, with vanilla frosting	1/6 pkg.	220
*Cinnamon (Pillsbury)		
Streusel Swirl	1/16 of cake	260
Coconut pecan (Betty Crocker)		
Snackin' Cake	1/9 of pkg.	190
Coffee cake:		
*(Aunt Jemima)	1/8 of cake	170
*(Pillsbury):		
Apple cinnamon	1/8 of cake	240
Cinnamon streusel	1/8 of cake	250
Date nut (Betty Crocker)		
Snackin' Cake	1/9 of pkg.	190
*(Pillsbury):		
Bundt:		
Fudge nut crown	1/16 of cake	220
Fudge, tunnel	1/16 of cake	270
Macaroon	1/16 of cake	250
Pillsbury Plus:		

Food and Description	Measure or Quantity	Calories
Fudge, dark	1/12 of cake	260
Fudge, marble	1/12 of cake	270
Streusel Swirl, German	1/16 of cake	260
Devil's food:		
*(Betty Crocker) *Supermoist*	1/12 of cake	260
(Duncan Hines) deluxe	1/12 of pkg.	190
*(Pillsbury) *Pillsbury Plus*	1/12 of cake	250
Fudge (See Chocolate)		
Golden chocolate chip		
(Betty Crocker) *Snackin' Cake*	1/9 pkg.	190
Lemon:		
(Betty Crocker):		
*Chiffon	1/12 of cake	190
Stir 'N Frost, with lemon		
frosting	1/12 pkg.	230
Supermoist	1/12 of cake	260
*(Pillsbury):		
Bundt, tunnel of	1/16 of cake	270
Streusel Swirl	1/16 of cake	260
*Lemon blueberry (Pillsbury)		
Bundt	1/16 of cake	200
Marble:		
*(Betty Crocker) *Supermoist*	1/12 of cake	260
*(Pillsbury):		
Bundt, supreme, ring	1/16 of cake	250
Streusel Swirl, fudge	1/16 of cake	260
*Oats'n brown sugar (Pillsbury)		
Pillsbury Plus	1/12 of cake	260
*Pecan brown sugar (Pillsbury)		
Streusel Swirl	1/16 of cake	260
*Orange (Betty Crocker)		
Supermoist	1/12 of cake	260
Pound:		
*(Betty Crocker) golden	1/12 of cake	200
*(Dromedary)	3/4" slice	210
*(Pillsbury) *Bundt*	1/16 of cake	230
Spice (Betty Crocker):		
Snackin' Cake, raisin	1/9 pkg.	180
Supermoist	1/12 of cake	260
Strawberry:		
*(Betty Crocker) *Supermoist*	1/12 of cake	260
*(Pillsbury) *Pillsbury Plus*	1/12 of cake	260
*Upside down (Betty Crocker)		
pineapple	1/9 of cake	270
White:		
*(Betty Crocker):		

Food and Description	Measure or Quantity	Calories
Stir 'N Frost, with chocolate frosting	⅙ of cake	220
Supermoist	½12 of cake	230
(Duncan Hines) deluxe	½12 of pkg.	188
*(Pillsbury) Pillsbury Plus	½12 of cake	240
Yellow:		
*(Betty Crocker) Supermoist	½12 of cake	260
(Duncan Hines) deluxe	½12 of pkg.	188
*(Pillsbury) Pillsbury Plus	½12 of cake	260
*Dietetic (Dia-Mel; Estee)	½10 of cake	100
CAMPARI, 45 proof	1 fl. oz.	66
CANDY, REGULAR:		
Almond, chocolate covered (Hershey's) Golden Almond	1 oz.	163
Almond, Jordan (Banner)	1¼-oz. box	154
Apricot Delight (Sahadi)	1 oz.	100
Baby Ruth	1.8-oz. piece	260
Butterfinger	1.6-oz. bar	220
Butterscotch Skimmers (Nabisco)	1 piece	25
Caramel:		
Caramel Flipper (Wayne)	1 oz.	128
Caramel Nip (Pearson)	1 piece	29
Charleston Chew	1½-oz. bar	179
Cherry, chocolate-covered (Nabisco; Welch's)	1 piece	67
Chocolate bar:		
Crunch (Nestlé)	1 1/16-oz. bar.	159
Milk:		
(Hershey's)	1.2-oz. bar	187
(Hershey's)	4-oz. bar	623
(Nestlé)	.35-oz. bar	53
(Nestlé)	1 1/16-oz. bar	159
Special Dark (Hershey's)	1.05-oz. bar	160
Special Dark (Hershey's)	4-oz. bar	611
Chocolate bar with almonds:		
(Hershey's) milk	.35-oz bar	55
(Hershey's) milk	1.15-oz. bar	180
(Nestlé)	1-oz.	150
Chocolate Parfait (Pearson)	1 piece	31
Chuckles	1 oz.	92
Clark Bar	1.4-oz. bar	188
Cluster, peanut, chocolate-covered (Hoffman)	1 cluster	205
Coffee Nip (Pearson)	1 piece	29
Coffioca (Pearson)	1 piece	31
Crispy Bar (Clark)	1¼-oz. bar	187

Food and Description	Measure or Quantity	Calories
Crows (Mason)	1 piece	11
Dots (Mason)	1 piece	11
Dutch Treat Bar (Clark)	1 1/16-oz. bar	160
Fudge (Nabisco) bar, *Home Style*	1 bar	90
Good & Plenty	1 oz.	100
Halvah (Sahadi) original and marble	1 oz.	150
Hollywood	1 1/2-oz. bar	185
Jelly bean (Curtiss)	1 piece	12
Jelly rings, *Chuckles*	1 piece	37
Jujubes, Chuckles	1 piece	13
Ju Jus:		
Assorted	1 piece	7
Coins or raspberries	1 piece	15
Kisses (Hershey's)	1 piece	27
Kit Kat	.6-oz. bar	80
Krackel Bar	.35-oz. bar	52
Krackel Bar	1.2-oz. bar	178
Licorice:		
Licorice Nips (Pearson)	1 piece	29
(Switzer) bars, bites or stix:		
Black	1 oz.	94
Cherry or strawberry	1 oz.	98
Chocolate	1 oz.	97
Twist:		
Black (American Licorice Co.)	1 piece	27
Black (Curtiss)	1 piece	27
Red (American Licorice Co.)	1 piece	33
Life Savers, drop	1 piece	10
Life Savers, mint	1 piece	7
Lollipops (Life Savers)	.9-oz. pop	99
Mallo Cup (Boyer)	9/16-oz. piece	54
Malted milk balls (Brach's)	1 piece	9
Mars Bar (M&M/Mars)	1.7-oz. bar	233
Marshmallow (Campfire)	1 oz.	111
Mary Jane (Miller):		
Small size	1.4 oz.	19
Large size	1 1/2-oz. bar	110
Milk Duds (Clark)	3/4-oz. box	89
Milky Way (M&M/Mars)	2.5-oz. bar	267
Mint or peppermint:		
After dinner (Richardson):		
Jelly center	1 oz.	104
Regular	1 oz.	109
Chocolate covered (Richardson)	1 oz.	106
Jamaica or Liberty Mints (Nabisco)	1 piece	24
Junior mint pattie (Nabisco)	1 piece	10
Mint Parfait (Pearson)	1 piece	31

Food and Description	Measure or Quantity	Calories
Peppermint Pattie (Nabisco)	1 piece	64
M & M's:		
Peanut	1.67-oz. pkg.	242
Plain	1.69-oz. pkg.	236
Mr. Goodbar (Hershey's)	.35-oz. bar	54
Mr. Goodbar (Hershey's)	1½-oz. bar	233
$100,000 Bar (Nestlé)	1¼-oz. bar	175
Orange slices (Curtiss)	1 piece	29
Peanut, chocolate-covered:		
(Curtiss)	1 piece	5
(Nabisco)	1 piece	24
Peanut crunch (Sahadi)	¾-oz. bar	110
Peanut, French burnt (Curtiss)	1 piece	4
Peanut brittle (Planters):		
Jumbo Peanut Block Bar	1 oz.	119
Jumbo Peanut Block Bar	1 piece (4 grams)	61
Peanut butter cup:		
(Boyer)	1.5-oz. pkg.	148
(Reese's)	.6-oz. cup	92
Raisin, chocolate-covered:		
(Nabisco)	1 piece	4
Raisinets (BB)	1 oz.	140
Reggie Bar	2-oz. bar	290
Rolo (Hershey's)	1 piece	30
Royals, mint chocolate		
(M&M/Mars)	1.52-oz. pkg.	212
Sesame Crunch (Sahadi)	¾-oz. bar	110
Snickers	2-oz. bar	275
Spearmint leaves (Curtiss)	1 piece	32
Starburst (M&M/Mars)	1-oz. serving	118
Sugar Babies (Nabisco)	1 piece	6
Sugar Daddy (Nabisco):		
Caramel sucker	1 piece	121
Nugget	1 piece	27
Sugar Mama (Nabisco)	1 piece	101
Summit bar (M&M/Mars)	1 oz.	144
Taffy:		
Salt water (Brach's)	1 piece	31
Turkish (Bonomo)	1 oz.	108
3 Musketeers	.8-oz. bar	99
3 Musketeers	2-oz. serving	255
Tootsie Roll:		
Chocolate	.23-oz. midgee	26
Chocolate	1/16-oz. bar	72
Chocolate	1-oz. bar	115
Flavored	.6-oz. square	19
Pop, all flavors	.49-oz. pop	55
Pop drop, all flavors	4.7-gram piece	19

Food and Description	Measure or Quantity	Calories
Twix, cookie bar (M&M/Mars)	1¾-oz. serving	246
Twix, peanut butter cookie bar (M&M/Mars)	1¾-oz. serving	261
Twizzlers:		
Cherry, chocolate, or strawberry	1 oz.	100
Licorice	1 oz.	90
Whatchamacallit (Hershey's)	1.15-oz. bar	176
World Series Bar	1 oz.	128
Zagnut Bar (Clark)	.7-oz. bar	92
CANDY, DIETETIC:		
Carob bar, *Joan's Natural:*		
Coconut	3-oz. bar	516
Fruit & nut	3-oz. bar	559
Honey bran	3-oz. bar	487
Peanut	3-oz. bar	521
Chocolate or chocolate-flavored bar: (Estee):		
Coconut, fruit & nut, milk, or toasted bran	.2-oz. square	30
Crunch	.2-oz. square	22
(Louis Sherry) coffee or orange flavored	.2-oz. square	22
Estee-ets, with peanuts (Estee)	1 piece	7
Gum drops (Estee) any flavor	1 piece	3
Hard candy:		
(Estee) assorted fruit	1 piece	11
(Louis Sherry)	1 piece	12
Mint:		
(Estee)	1 piece	4
(Sunkist):		
Mini mint	1 piece	1
Roll mint	1 piece	4
Peanut butter cup (Estee)	1 cup	45
Raisins, chocolate-covered (Estee)	1 piece	5
CANNELLONI, frozen:		
(Stouffer's) beef & pork with mornay sauce	9⅝-oz. pkg.	240
(Weight Watchers) one-compartment	13-oz. meal	450
CANTALOUPE, cubed	½ cup (3 oz.)	24
CAPERS (Crosse & Blackwell)	1 tsp.	2
CAP'N CRUNCH, cereal (Quaker):		
Regular	¾ cup	121
Crunchberry	¾ cup	120
Peanut butter	¾ cup	127
CAPOCOLLO (Hormel)	1 oz.	80
CARAWAY SEED (French's)	1 tsp.	8

28

Food and Description	Measure or Quantity	Calories
CARNATION INSTANT BREAKFAST:		
Bar:		
Chocolate chip	1 bar	200
Peanut butter crunch	1 bar	180
Packets, all flavors	1 packet	130
CARROT:		
Raw	5½″ × 1″ piece	21
Boiled, slices	½ cup	24
Canned, regular pack, solids & liq.:		
(Del Monte) sliced or whole	½ cup	30
(Libby's)	½ cup	20
Canned, dietetic pack, solids & liq., (S&W) *Nutradiet*, green label	½ cup	30
Frozen:		
(Birds Eye) whole, baby deluxe	⅓ pkg.	84
(Green Giant) cuts, in butter sauce	½ cup	80
(Seabrook Farms)	⅓ pkg.	39
CASABA MELON	1-lb. melon	61
CASHEW NUT:		
(Fisher):		
Dry roasted	1 oz.	156
Oil roasted	1 oz.	159
(Planters):		
Dry roasted	1 oz.	160
Oil roasted	1 oz.	170
CATSUP:		
Regular:		
(Del Monte)	1 T.	17
(Smucker's)	1 T.	21
Dietetic or low calorie:		
(Del Monte) No Salt Added	1 T.	15
(Featherweight)	1 T.	6
CAULIFLOWER:		
Raw or boiled buds	½ cup	14
Frozen:		
(Birds Eye) regular or florets, deluxe	⅓ of pkg.	28
(Green Giant) in cheese sauce	½ cup	60
CAVIAR:		
Pressed	1 oz.	90
Whole eggs	1 T.	42
CELERY:		
1 large outer stalk	8″ × 1½″ at root end	7
Diced or cut	½ cup	9
Salt (French's)	1 tsp.	12
Seed (French's)	1 tsp.	11

Food and Description	Measure or Quantity	Calories
CERTS	1 piece	61
CERVELAT (Hormel) Viking	1-oz. serving	90
CHABLIS WINE:		
(Almaden) light	3 fl. oz.	42
(Louis M. Martini)	3 fl. oz.	59
(Paul Masson):		
Regular	3 fl. oz.	71
Light	3 fl. oz.	45
CHAMPAGNE:		
(Bollinger)	3 fl. oz.	72
(Great Western):		
Regular	3 fl. oz.	71
Brut	3 fl. oz.	74
Pink	3 fl. oz.	81
(Taylor) dry	3 fl. oz.	78
CHARDONNAY WINE		
(Louis M. Martini)	3 fl. oz.	61
CHARLOTTE RUSSE, homemade recipe	4 oz.	324
CHEERIOS, cereal, regular or honey & nut	1 oz.	110
CHEESE:		
American or cheddar:		
Cube, natural	1" cube	68
Laughing Cow, natural	1 oz.	110
(Sargento):		
Midget, regular or sharp	1 oz.	114
Shredded, non-dairy	1 oz.	90
Wispride	1 oz.	115
Blue:		
(Frigo)	1 oz.	100
(Sargento) cold pack or crumbled	1 oz.	100
Bonbino, Laughing Cow, natural	1 oz.	103
Brick (Sargento)	1 oz.	105
Brie (Sargento) Danish Danko	1 oz.	80
Burgercheese (Sargento) Danish Danko	1 oz.	106
Camembert (Sargento) Danish Danko	1 oz.	88
Colby:		
(Featherweight) low sodium	1 oz.	100
(Pauly) low sodium	1 oz.	115
(Sargento) shredded or sliced	1 oz.	112
Cottage:		
Unflavored:		
(Bison):		
Regular	1 oz.	29
Dietetic	1 oz.	22

Food and Description	Measure or Quantity	Calories
(Dairylea)	1 oz.	30
(Friendship)	1 oz.	30
Flavored (Friendship) Dutch apple	1 oz.	31
Cream, plain, unwhipped:		
(Friendship)	1 oz.	103
(Frigo)	1 oz.	100
Edam:		
(House of Gold)	1 oz.	100
Laughing Cow	1 oz.	100
Farmers:		
Dutch Garden Brand	1 oz.	100
(Friendship) regular or no salt added	1 oz.	40
(Sargento)	1 oz.	72
Wispride	1 oz.	100
Feta (Sargento) Danish, cups	1 oz.	76
Gjetost (Sargento) Norwegian	1 oz.	118
Gouda:		
Laughing Cow	1 oz.	110
(Sargento) baby, caraway or smoked	1 oz.	101
Wispride	1 oz.	100
Gruyère, *Swiss Knight*	1 oz.	100
Havarti (Sargento):		
Creamy	1 oz.	90
Creamy, 60% mild	1 oz.	117
Hoop (Friendship) natural	1 oz.	21
Hot pepper (Sargento)	1 oz.	112
Jarlsberg (Sargento) Norwegian	1 oz.	100
Kettle Moraine (Sargento)	1 oz.	100
Limburger (Sargento) natural	1 oz.	93
Monterey Jack:		
(Frigo)	1 oz.	100
Sargento) midget, Longhorn, shredded or sliced	1 oz.	106
Mozzarella:		
(Fisher) part skim milk	1 oz.	90
(Sargento):		
Bar, rounds, shredded regular or with spices, sliced for pizzas or square	1 oz.	79
Whole milk	1 oz.	100
Muenster:		
(Sargento) red rind	1 oz.	104
Wispride	1 oz.	100
Nibblin Curds (Sargento)	1 oz.	114

31

Food and Description	Measure or Quantity	Calories
Parmesan:		
(Frigo):		
Grated	1 T.	23
Whole	1 oz.	110
(Sargento):		
Grated	1 T.	27
Wedge	1 oz.	110
Pizza (Sargento) shredded or sliced	1 oz.	90
Pot (Sargento) regular, French onion or garlic	1 oz.	30
Provolone:		
(Frigo)	1 oz.	90
Laughing Cow:		
Cube	⅙ oz.	12
Wedge	¾ oz.	55
(Sargento) sliced	1 oz.	100
Ricotta:		
(Frigo) part skim milk	1 oz.	43
(Sargento):		
Part skim milk	1 oz.	39
Whole milk	1 oz.	49
Romano (Sargento) wedge	1 oz.	110
Roquefort, natural	1 oz.	104
Samsoe (Sargento) Danish	1 oz.	79
Scamorze (Frigo)	1 oz.	79
Semisoft, Laughing Cow:		
Babybel	1 oz.	91
Bonbel	1 oz.	99
Stirred curd (Frigo)	1 oz.	110
String (Sargento)	1 oz.	90
Swiss:		
(Fisher) natural	1 oz.	100
(Frigo) domestic	1 oz.	100
(Sargento) domestic or Finland, sliced	1 oz.	107
Taco (Sargento) shredded	1 oz.	105
Washed curd (Frigo)	1 oz.	110
CHEESE FONDUE, *Swiss Knight*	1 oz.	110
CHEESE FOOD:		
American or cheddar:		
(Fisher) *Ched-O-Mate* or *Sandwich-Mate*	1 oz.	90
(Weight Watchers) colored or white	1-oz. slice	50
Wispride:		
Regular	1 oz.	90
& blue cheese	1 oz.	100
Hickory smoked	1 oz.	90

32

& port wine	1 oz.	100
Sharp	1 oz.	90
Cheez-ola (Fisher)	1 oz.	90
Chef's Delight (Fisher)	1 oz.	70
Count Down (Pauly)	1 oz.	40
Cracker snack (Sargento)	1 oz.	90
Loaf, *Count Down* (Pauly)	1 oz.	100
Mun-chee (Pauly)	1 oz.	100
Pimiento (Pauly)	.8-oz. slice	73
Pizza-Mate (Fisher)	1 oz.	90
Swiss (Pauly)	.8-oz. slice	74
CHEESE PUFFS, frozen (Durkee)	1 piece	59
CHEESE SPREAD:		
American or cheddar:		
(Fisher)	1 oz.	80
Laughing Cow	1 oz.	73
(Nabisco) *Snack Mate*	1 tsp.	16
Blue, *Laughing Cow*	1 oz.	72
Cheese'n Bacon (Nabisco)		
Snack Mate	1 tsp.	16
Cheese Whiz (Kraft)	1 oz.	.78
Gruyère, *Laughing Cow, La Vache*		
Que Rit	1 oz.	72
Pimiento:		
(Nabisco) *Snack Mate*	1 tsp.	15
(Price')	1 oz.	80
Provolone, *Laughing Cow*	1 oz.	72
Sharp (Pauly)	.8 oz.	77
Swiss, process (Pauly)	.8 oz.	76
Velveeta (Kraft)	1 oz.	85
CHEESE STRAW, frozen (Durkee)	1 piece	29
CHENIN BLANC WINE		
(Louis M. Martini)	3 fl. oz.	60
CHERRY, sweet:		
Fresh, with stems	½ cup	41
Canned, regular pack (Del Monte)		
dark, solids & liq.	½ cup	50
Canned, dietetic, solids & liq.:		
(Diet Delight) with pits,		
water pack	½ cup	70
(Featherweight) dark, water pack	½ cup	60
CHERRY, CANDIED	1 oz.	96
CHERRY DRINK:		
Canned:		
(Hi-C)	6 fl. oz.	93
(Lincoln) cherry berry	6 fl. oz.	100
*Mix (Hi-C)	6 fl. oz.	72

Food and Description	Measure or Quantity	Calories
CHERRY HEERING		
(Hiram Walker)	1 fl. oz.	80
CHERRY JELLY:		
Sweetened (Smucker's)	1 T.	53
Dietetic:		
(Dia-Mel)	1 T.	6
(Featherweight)	1 T.	16
CHERRY LIQUEUR (DeKuyper)	1 fl. oz.	75
CHERRY PRESERVES OR JAM:		
Sweetened (Smucker's)	1 T.	53
Dietetic (Dia-Mel)	1 T.	6
CHESTNUT, fresh, in shell	¼ lb.	220
CHEWING GUM:		
Sweetened:		
Bazooka, bubble	1 slice	18
Beechies, Chiclets, tiny size	1 piece	6
Beech Nut; Beeman's Big Red; Black Jack; Clove; Doublemint; Freedent; Fruit Punch; Juicy Fruit, Spearmint (Wrigley's); *Teaberry*	1 stick	10
Dentyne	1 piece	4
Hubba Bubba (Wrigley's)	1 piece	23
Dietetic:		
(Clark; *Care*Free*)	1 piece	7
(Estee) bubble or regular	1 piece	5
(Featherweight) bubble or regular	1 piece	4
Orbit (Wrigley's)	1 piece	8
CHEX, cereal (Ralston Purina):		
Rice	1 cup	110
Wheat	⅔ cup	110
Wheat & raisins	¾ cup	130
CHIANTI WINE:		
(Italian Swiss Colony)	3 fl. oz.	83
(Louis M. Martini)	3 fl. oz.	90
CHICKEN:		
Broiler, cooked, meat only	3 oz.	116
Fryer, fried, meat & skin	3 oz.	212
Fryer, fried, meat only	3 oz.	178
Fryer, fried, a 2½-lb. chicken (weighed with bone before cooking) will give you:		
Back	1 back	139
Breast	½ breast	160
Leg or drumstick	1 leg	87
Neck	1 neck	127
Rib	1 rib	41

Food and Description	Measure or Quantity	Calories
Thigh	1 thigh	122
Wing	1 wing	82
Fried skin	1 oz.	119
Hen & cock:		
Stewed, meat & skin	3 oz.	269
Stewed, dark meat only	3 oz.	176
Stewed, light meat only	3 oz.	153
Stewed, diced	½ cup	139
Roaster, roasted, dark or light meat, without skin	3 oz.	156
CHICKEN À LA KING:		
Home recipe	1 cup	468
Canned (Swanson)	½ of 10½-oz. can	180
Frozen:		
(Banquet) *Cookin' Bag*	5-oz. pkg.	138
(Green Giant) twin pouch, with biscuits	9-oz. entree	370
(Stouffer's) with rice	9½-oz. pkg.	330
(Weight Watchers)	9-oz. pkg.	230
CHICKEN BOUILLON:		
(Herb-Ox):		
Cube	1 cube	6
Packet	1 packet	12
Low Sodium (Featherweight)	1 tsp.	18
CHICKEN, BONED, CANNED:		
Regular:		
(Hormel) chunk, breast	6¾-oz. serving	350
(Swanson) chunk:		
Mixin' chicken	2½ oz.	130
White	2½ oz.	110
Low sodium (Featherweight)	2½ oz.	154
CHICKEN, CREAMED, frozen (Stouffer's)	6½ oz.	300
CHICKEN DINNER OR ENTREE:		
Canned (Swanson) & dumplings	7½ oz.	220
Frozen:		
(Banquet):		
American Favorites	11-oz. dinner	359
Extra Helping:		
& dressing	19-oz. dinner	808
Fried	17-oz. dinner	744
(Green Giant):		
Baked:		
In BBQ sauce with corn on the cob	1 meal	350
Stir fry and garden vegetables	10-oz. entree	250

Food and Description	Measure or Quantity	Calories
Twin pouch, & broccoli, with rice in cheese sauce	9½-oz. entree	330
(Morton):		
Regular:		
Boneless	10-oz. dinner	222
Sliced	5-oz. pkg.	130
Country Table, fried	15-oz. entree	710
King Size, fried	17-oz. dinner	860
(Stouffer's):		
Regular:		
Cacciatore, with spaghetti	11¼-oz. meal	313
Divan	8½-oz. serving	336
Lean Cuisine:		
Glazed with vegetable rice	8½-oz. serving	270
& vegetables with vermicelli	12¾-oz. serving	260
(Swanson):		
Regular, in white wine sauce	8¼-oz. entree	350
Hungry Man:		
Boneless	19-oz. dinner	680
Fried:		
White portion	15¼-oz. dinner	950
White portion with whipped potato	11¾-oz. entree	720
TV Brand, fried:		
Barbecue	11¼-oz. dinner	570
Nibbles, with french fries	6-oz. entree	590
3-course, fried	15-oz. dinner	590
(Weight Watchers):		
Cacciatore	10-oz. serving	290
Oriental style	12-oz. serving	251
Parmigiana, 2-compartment	7¾-oz. serving	220
Sliced in celery sauce, 2-compartment	8½-oz. serving	207
Southern fried patty, 2-compartment	9½-oz. serving	220
CHICKEN, FRIED, frozen:		
(Banquet)	2-lb. pkg.	2591
(Morton)	2-lb. pkg.	1490
(Swanson):		
Assorted	3¼-oz. serving	290
Breast portions	3¼-oz. serving	250
Nibbles	3¼-oz. serving	300
Take-out style	3¼-oz. serving	270
CHICKEN & NOODLES, frozen:		
(Green Giant) twin pouch, with vegetables	9-oz. pkg.	365
(Stouffer's):		
Escalloped	5¾-oz. serving	252
Paprikash	10½-oz. serving	391

Food and Description	Measure or Quantity	Calories
CHICKEN NUGGETS, frozen		
(Banquet)	12-oz. pkg.	932
CHICKEN, PACKAGED		
(Louis Rich) breast, oven roasted	1-oz. slice	40
CHICKEN PATTY, frozen (Banquet)	12-oz. pkg.	900
CHICKEN PIE, frozen:		
(Banquet) regular	8-oz. pie	427
(Morton)	8-oz. pie	345
(Stouffer's)	10-oz. pie	493
(Swanson) regular	8-oz. pie	420
(Van de Kamp's)	7½-oz. pie	520
CHICKEN PUFF, frozen (Durkee)	½-oz. piece	49
CHICKEN SALAD (Carnation)	¼ of 7½-oz. can	94
CHICKEN SOUP (See SOUP, chicken)		
CHICKEN SPREAD:		
(Hormel)	1 oz.	60
(Underwood) chunky	½ of 4¾-oz. can	63
CHICKEN STEW, canned:		
Regular:		
(Libby's) with dumplings	8 oz.	194
(Swanson)	7⅜ oz.	170
Dietetic (Dia-Mel)	8-oz. serving	150
CHICKEN STOCK BASE (French's)	1 tsp.	8
CHICK-FIL-A:		
Sandwich	5.4-oz. serving	404
Soup, hearty; breast of chicken:		
Small	8⅓ oz.	131
Large	14.3 oz.	230
CHICK'N QUICK, frozen (Tyson):		
Breast fillet	3 oz.	210
Breast pattie	3 oz.	240
Chick'N Cheddar	3 oz.	250
Cordon bleu	5 oz.	300
Kiev	5 oz.	410
Swiss'N Bacon	3 oz.	260
CHILI OR CHILI CON CARNE:		
Canned, regular pack:		
Beans only:		
(Hormel)	5 oz.	130
(Van Camp) Mexican style	1 cup	250
With beans:		
(Hormel) regular or hot	7½-oz. serving	310
(Libby's)	7½-oz. serving	270
(Swanson)	7¾-oz. serving	310
Without beans:		

Food and Description	Measure or Quantity	Calories
(Hormel) regular or hot	7½-oz. serving	370
(Libby's)	7½ oz.	390
Canned, dietetic pack:		
(Dia-Mel) with beans	8-oz. serving	360
(Featherweight) with beans	7½ oz.	270
Frozen, with beans (Stouffer's)		
	8¾-oz. pkg.	270
CHILI SAUCE:		
(Del Monte)	¼ cup (2 oz.)	70
(Ortega) green	1 oz.	6
(Featherweight) Dietetic	1 T.	8
CHILI SEASONING MIX:		
*(Durkee)	1 cup	465
(French's) *Chili-O*	1¾-oz. pkg.	150
(McCormick)	1.2-oz. pkg.	106
CHOCO-DILE (Hostess)	2-oz. piece	235
CHOCOLATE, BAKING:		
(Baker's):		
Bitter or unsweetened	1 oz.	180
Semi-sweet, chips	½ cup	207
Sweetened, *German's*	1 oz.	158
(Hershey's):		
Bitter or unsweetened	1 oz.	188
Sweetened:		
Dark chips, regular or mini	1 oz.	151
Milk, chips	1 oz.	148
Semi-sweet, chips	1 oz.	150
(Nestlé):		
Bitter or unsweetened, *Choco-bake*	1-oz. packet	180
Sweet or semi-sweet, morsels	1 oz.	150
CHOCOLATE ICE CREAM (See ICE CREAM, Chocolate)		
CHOCOLATE SYRUP (See SYRUP, Chocolate)		
CHOP SUEY, frozen (Stouffer's) beef with rice	12-oz. pkg.	355
***CHOP SUEY SEASONING MIX** (Durkee)	1¾ cups	557
CHOWDER (See SOUP, Chowder)		
CHOW MEIN:		
Canned:		
(Hormel) Pork, *Short Orders*	7½-oz. can	140
(La Choy):		
Regular:		
Beef	1 cup	72
Chicken	½ of 1-lb. can	68

Food and Description	Measure or Quantity	Calories
Meatless	1 cup	47
Shrimp	1 cup	61
*Bi-pack:		
Beef or vegetable	¾ cup	60
Beef pepper oriental, chicken or shrimp	¾ cup	70
Pork	¾ cup	90
Frozen:		
(Green Giant) chicken	9-oz. entree	215
(La Choy):		
Chicken	11-oz. dinner	356
Shrimp	11-oz. dinner	323
(Stouffer's) *Lean Cuisine*, with rice	11¼-oz. serving	240
CHOW MEIN SEASONING MIX (Kikkoman)	1⅛-oz. pkg.	98
CHUTNEY (Major Grey's)	1 T.	53
CINNAMON, GROUND (French's)	1 tsp.	6
CITRUS COOLER DRINK, canned (Hi-C)	6 fl. oz.	93
CLAM:		
Raw, all kinds, meat only	1 cup (8 oz.)	186
Raw, soft, meat & liq.	1 lb. (weighed in shell)	142
Canned (Doxsee):		
Chopped & minced, solids & liq.	4 oz.	59
Chopped, meat only	4 oz.	111
Frozen:		
(Howard Johnson's)	5-oz. pkg.	395
(Mrs. Paul's) fried, light	2½-oz. serving	230
CLAMATO COCKTAIL (Mott's)	6 fl. oz.	80
CLAM JUICE (Snow)	½ cup	15
CLARET WINE:		
(Gold Seal)	3 fl. oz.	82
(Taylor) 12.5% alcohol	3 fl. oz.	72
CLORETS, gum or mint	1 piece	6
COBBLER, frozen		
(Weight Watchers)	4-oz. serving	160
COCOA:		
Dry, unsweetened:		
(Hershey's)	1 T.	29
(Sultana)	1 T.	30
(Alba '66) instant, all flavors	1 envelope	60
(Carnation) all flavors	1-oz. pkg.	110
(Hershey's):		
Hot	1 oz.	110
Instant	3 T.	76
(Nestlé) With mini marshmallows	1 oz.	110

Food and Description	Measure or Quantity	Calories
(Ovaltine) hot 'n rich	1 oz.	120
*Swiss Miss, regular or with mini marshmallows	6 fl. oz.	110
Mix, dietetic:		
(Carnation):		
70 Calorie	¾-oz. packet	70
*Sugar free	6 fl. oz.	50
*(Featherweight)	6 fl. oz.	50
Swiss Miss, instant, lite	3 T.	70
COCOA KRISPIES, cereal		
(Kellogg's)	¾ cup	110
COCOA PUFFS, cereal		
(General Mills)	1 oz.	110
COCONUT:		
Fresh, meat only	2″ × 2″ × ½″ piece	156
Grated or shredded, loosely packed	½ cup	225
Dried:		
(Baker's):		
Angel Flake	⅓ cup	118
Cookie	⅓ cup	186
Premium shred	⅓ cup	138
(Durkee) shredded	¼ cup	69
COCO WHEATS, cereal	1 T.	44
COD:		
Broiled	3 oz.	145
Frozen (Van de Kamp's)		
Today's Catch	4-oz. serving	80
COFFEE:		
Regular:		
*Max-Pax; Maxwell House Electra Perk; Yuban, Yuban Electra Matic	6 fl. oz.	2
*Mellow Roast	6 fl. oz.	8
Decaffeinated:		
*Brim, regular or electric perk	6 fl. oz.	2
*Brim, freeze-dried; Decafé; Nescafé	6 fl. oz.	4
*Sanka, regular or electric perk	6 fl. oz.	2
Instant:		
*Mellow Roast	6 fl. oz.	8
*Sunrise	6 fl. oz.	6
*Mix (General Foods)		
International Coffee:		
Café Amaretto, Café Francais	6 fl. oz.	59
Café Vienna, Orange Capuccino	6 fl. oz.	65
Irish Mocha Mint	6 fl. oz.	55
Suisse Mocha	6 fl. oz.	58
COFFEE CAKE (See CAKE, Coffee)		

Food and Description	Measure or Quantity	Calories
COFFEE LIQUEUR (DeKuyper)	1½ fl. oz.	140
COFFEE SOUTHERN	1 fl. oz.	79
COLA SOFT DRINK (See SOFT DRINK, Cola)		
COLD DUCK WINE (Great Western) pink	3 fl. oz.	92
COLESLAW, solids & liq., made with mayonnaise-type salad dressing	1 cup	119
***COLESLAW MIX** (Libby's)		
Super Slaw	½ cup	240
COLLARDS:		
Leaves, cooked	⅓ pkg.	31
Canned (Sunshine) chopped, solids & liq.	½ cup	25
Frozen:		
(Birds Eye) chopped	⅓ pkg.	30
(McKenzie) chopped	⅓ pkg.	25
(Southland) chopped	⅓ of 16-oz. pkg.	30
COMPLETE CEREAL (Elam's)	1 oz.	109
CONCORD WINE:		
(Gold Seal)	3 fl. oz.	125
(Pleasant Valley) red	3 fl. oz.	90
COOKIE, REGULAR:		
Almond Windmill (Nabisco)	1 piece	47
Animal:		
(Dixie Belle)	1 piece	8
(Keebler):		
Regular	1 piece	12
Iced	1 piece	24
(Nabisco) *Barnum's Animals*	1 piece	12
Apple (Pepperidge Farm)	1 piece	50
Apple Crisp (Nabisco)	1 piece	50
Apple Spice (Pepperidge Farm)	1 piece	53
Apricot Raspberry (Pepperidge Farm)	1 piece	50
Assortment:		
(Nabisco) *Mayfair:*		
Crown creme sandwich	1 piece	53
Fancy shortbread biscuit	1 piece	22
Filigree creme sandwich	1 piece	60
Mayfair creme sandwich	1 piece	65
Tea rose creme	1 piece	53
(Pepperidge Farm):		
Butter	1 piece	55
Champagne	1 piece	32
Chocolate lace & Pirouette	1 piece	37
Marseilles	1 piece	45

Food and Description	Measure or Quantity	Calories
Seville	1 piece	55
Southport	1 piece	75
Bordeaux (Pepperidge Farm)	1 piece	33
Brown edge wafer (Nabisco)	1 piece	28
Brownie:		
(Hostess)	1.25-oz. piece	157
(Pepperidge Farm) chocolate nut	.4-oz. piece	57
(Sara Lee) frozen	⅛ of 13-oz. pkg.	199
Brusseles (Pepperidge Farm)	1 piece	53
Brusseles Mint (Pepperidge Farm)	1 piece	67
Butter (Nabisco)	1 piece	23
Cappucino (Pepperidge Farm)	1 piece	53
Caramel peanut log (Nabisco)		
Heyday	1 piece	120
Chessman (Pepperidge Farm)	1 piece	43
Chocolate & chocolate-covered:		
(Nabisco):		
Pinwheel, cake	1 piece	140
Snap	1 piece	16
Chocolate chip:		
(Keebler) *Rich'N Chips*	1 piece	81
(Nabisco):		
Chips Ahoy!	1 piece	53
Chocolate	1 piece	53
(Pepperidge Farm):		
Regular size	1 piece	50
Large size	1 piece	130
Coconut:		
(Keebler) chocolate drop	1 piece	83
(Nabisco) bar, *Bakers Bonus*	1 piece	43
Coconut Granola		
(Pepperidge Farm)	1 piece	57
Date Nut Granola (Pepperidge Farm)	1 piece	53
Fig bar:		
(Keebler)	1 piece	74
(Nabisco):		
Fig Newtons	1 piece	60
Fig Wheats	1 piece	60
Gingerman (Pepperidge Farm)	1 piece	57
Gingersnaps (Nabisco) old fashioned	1 piece	30
Granola (Pepperidge Farm) large	1 piece	120
Hazelnut (Pepperidge Farm)	1 piece	57
Ladyfinger	3¼″ × 1⅜″ × 1⅛″	40
Lemon nut (Pepperidge Farm) large	1 piece	140
Lido (Pepperidge Farm)	1 piece	95
Macaroon, coconut (Nabisco)	1 piece	95

Food and Description	Measure or Quantity	Calories
Marshmallow:		
(Nabisco):		
Mallomars	1 piece	60
Puffs, cocoa covered	1 piece	85
Sandwich	1 piece	30
Twirls cakes	1 piece	130
(Planters) banana pie	1 oz.	127
Milano (Pepperidge Farm)	1 piece	60
Mint Milano (Pepperidge Farm)	1 piece	76
Molasses (Nabisco) *Pantry*	1 piece	60
Molasses Crisp (Pepperidge Farm)	1 piece	33
Nilla wafer (Nabisco)	1 piece	19
Oatmeal:		
(Keebler) old fashioned	1 piece	83
(Nabisco):		
Bakers Bonus	1 piece	80
(Pepperidge Farm):		
Irish	1 piece	47
Large	1 piece	120
Orange Milano (Pepperidge Farm)	1 piece	76
Peanut & peanut butter (Nabisco):		
Biscos	1 piece	47
Fudge	1 piece	50
Nutter Butter	1 piece	70
Peanut brittle (Nabisco)	1 piece	50
Pecan Sandies (Keebler)	1 piece	86
Raisin	1 oz.	107
Raisin (Nabisco) fruit biscuit	1 piece	60
Raisin bar (Keebler) iced	1 piece	80
Raisin Bran (Pepperidge Farm)	1 piece	53
Sandwich:		
(Keebler):		
Chocolate fudge	1 piece	83
Elfwich	1 piece	55
Pitter Patter	1 piece	83
(Nabisco):		
Cameo, creme	1 piece	70
Mystic mint	1 piece	90
Oreo	1 piece	50
Oreo, double stuff	1 piece	70
Vanilla, *Cookie Break*	1 piece	50
Shortbread or shortcake:		
(Nabisco):		
Cookie Little	1 piece	6
Lorna Doone	1 piece	40
Melt-A-Way	1 piece	70
Pecan	1 piece	80

Food and Description	Measure or Quantity	Calories
(Pepperidge Farm)	1 piece	75
Social Tea, biscuit (Nabisco)	1 piece	22
Spiced Windmill (Keebler)	1 piece	60
Sugar cookie (Nabisco) rings, *Bakers Bonus*	1 piece	70
Sugar wafer:		
(Dutch Twin) any flavor	1 piece	36
(Keebler) *Krisp Kreem*	1 piece	29
(Nabisco) *Biscos*	1 piece	19
Sunflower Raisin (Pepperidge Farm)	1 piece	53
Tahiti (Pepperidge Farm)	1 piece	85
Waffle creme (Dutch Twin)	1 piece	45
Zanzibar (Pepperidge Farm)	1 piece	40
COOKIE, DIETETIC (Estee):		
Chocolate Chip, coconut or oatmeal raisin	1 piece	28
Sandwich duplex	1 piece	47
Wafer, chocolate covered	1 piece	120
COOKIE CRISP, cereal, any flavor	1 cup	110
***COOKIE DOUGH:**		
Refrigerated (Pillsbury):		
Chocolate chip or sugar	1 cookie	57
Double chocolate or peanut butter	1 cookie	57
Frozen (Rich's):		
Chocolate chip	1 cookie	138
Oatmeal	1 cookie	125
***COOKIE MIX:**		
Regular:		
Brownie:		
(Betty Crocker):		
Fudge, regular size	¹⁄₁₆ of pan	150
Walnut, family size	¹⁄₂₄ of pan	130
(Nestlé)	¹⁄₂₃ of pkg.	150
(Pillsbury) fudge, regular size	2″ sq. (¹⁄₁₆ of pkg.)	150
Chocolate chip:		
(Betty Crocker) *Big Batch*	1 cookie	60
(Duncan Hines)	¹⁄₃₆ of pkg.	72
(Nestlé)	1 cookie	60
(Quaker)	1 cookie	75
Fudge chip (Quaker)	1 cookie	75
Macaroon, coconut (Betty Crocker)	¹⁄₂₄ of pkg.	80
Oatmeal:		
(Betty Crocker) *Big Batch*	1 cookie	65
(Quaker)	1 cookie	66
Peanut butter (Duncan Hines)	¹⁄₃₆ pkg.	68

44

Food and Description	Measure or Quantity	Calories
Sugar:		
(Betty Crocker) *Big Batch*	1 cookie	60
(Duncan Hines) golden	1 cookie	59
Dietetic (Estee) brownie	2″ × 2″ sq. cookie	45
COOKING SPRAY, *Mazola No Stick*	2-second spray	8
CORN:		
Fresh, on the cob, boiled	5″ × 1¾″ ear	70
Canned, regular pack, solids & liq.		
(Del Monte):		
Cream style, golden	½ cup	95
Whole kernel	½ cup	100
(Green Giant):		
Ceam style	4¼ oz.	96
Whole kernel, golden	4¼ oz.	79
Whole kernel, *Mexicorn*	3½ oz.	90
(Le Sueur) whole kernel	4¼ oz.	80
(Libby's) cream style	½ cup	100
(Stokely-Van Camp):		
Cream style	½ cup	105
Whole kernel, solids & liq.	½ cup	74
Canned, dietetic, pack, solids & liq.:		
(Del Monte) No Salt Added	½ cup	90
(Diet Delight)	½ cup	60
(S&W) *Nutradiet,* whole kernel, green label	½ cup	80
Frozen:		
(Birds Eye):		
On the cob:		
Farmside	4.4-oz. ear	140
Little Ears	2.3-oz. ear	73
With butter sauce	⅓ of pkg.	98
(Green Giant):		
On the cob:		
Nibbler	2.7-oz. ear	80
Niblet Ear	4.9-oz. ear	140
Whole kernel, *Harvest Fresh*	½ cup	101
Whole kernel, *Niblets,* golden, polybag	⅓ of pkg.	80
(Seabrook Farms):		
On the cob	5″ ear	140
Whole kernel	⅓ of pkg.	97
CORNBREAD:		
Home recipe:		
Corn pone	4 oz.	231
Spoon bread	4 oz.	221
*Mix:		
(Aunt Jemima)	⅙ of pkg.	220

Food and Description	Measure or Quantity	Calories
(Dromedary)	2" × 2" piece	130
(Pillsbury) *Ballard*	⅛ of recipe	140
*CORN DOGS, frozen:		
(Hormel)	1 piece	220
(Oscar Mayer)	1 piece	328
CORNED BEEF:		
Cooked, boneless, medium fat	4-oz. serving	422
Canned, regular pack:		
Dinty Moore (Hormel)	2-oz. serving	130
(Libby's)	⅓ of 7-oz. can	160
Canned, dietetic (Featherweight) loaf	2½-oz. serving	90
Packaged (Eckrich) sliced	1-oz. slice	41
CORNED BEEF HASH, CANNED:		
(Libby's)	⅓ of 24-oz. can	420
Mary Kitchen (Hormel)	7½-oz. serving	360
CORNED BEEF HASH DINNER, frozen (Banquet)	10-oz. dinner	372
CORNED BEEF SPREAD (Underwood)	½ of 4½-oz. can	120
CORN FLAKE CRUMBS (Kellogg's)	¼ cup	110
CORN FLAKES, cereal:		
(General Mills) *Country*	1 cup	110
(Kellogg's) regular	1 cup	110
(Ralston Purina) regular	1 cup	110
CORN MEAL:		
Bolted (Aunt Jemima/Quaker)	3 T.	102
Degermed	¼ cup	125
Mix, bolted (Aunt Jemima) white	1 cup	392
CORNSTARCH (Argo; Kingsford's; Duryea)	1 tsp.	10
CORN SYRUP (See SYRUP, Corn)		
COUGH DROP:		
(Beech-Nut)	1 drop	10
(Pine Bros.)	1 drop	8
COUNT CHOCULA, cereal (General Mills)	1 oz. (1 cup)	110
CRAB:		
Fresh, steamed:		
Whole	½ lb.	101
Meat only	4 oz.	105
Canned, drained	4 oz.	115
Frozen (Wakefield's)	4 oz.	96
CRAB APPLE, flesh only	¼ lb.	71
CRAB APPLE JELLY (Smucker's)	1 T.	53
CRAB, DEVILED, frozen (Mrs. Paul's) breaded & fried	½ of 6-oz. pkg.	154

Food and Description	Measure or Quantity	Calories
CRAB IMPERIAL, home recipe	1 cup	323
CRACKER, PUFFS & CHIPS:		
Arrowroot biscuit (Nabisco)	1 piece	20
Bacon'n Dip (Nabisco)	1 piece	9
Bacon-flavored thins (Nabisco)	1 piece	11
Bacon Nips	1 oz.	147
Bacon toast (Keebler)	1 piece	16
Biscos (Nabisco)	1 piece	19
Bran wafer (Featherweight)	1 piece	13
Bugles (General Mills)	1 oz.	150
Cheese flavored:		
Cheddar triangles (Nabisco)	1 piece	9
Cheese'n Crunch (Nabisco)	1 oz.	160
Chee-Tos, crunchy or puffy	1 oz.	160
Cheez Balls (Planters)	1 oz.	160
Cheez Curls (Planters)	1 oz.	160
Country cheddar'n sesame		
(Nabisco)	1 piece	9
(Dixie Belle)	1 piece	6
Nacho cheese cracker (Keebler)	1 piece	11
Nips (Nabisco)	1 piece	5
Swiss cheese (Nabisco)	1 piece	10
Tid-Bit (Nabisco)	1 oz.	150
Chicken in a Biskit (Nabisco)	1 piece	11
Chippers (Nabisco)	1 piece	15
Chipsters (Nabisco)	1 piece	2
Club cracker (Keebler)	1 piece	15
Corn chips:		
(Bachman) regular or BBQ	1 oz.	150
(Featherweight) low sodium	1 oz.	170
Fritos:		
Regular	1 oz.	160
Barbecue flavor	1 oz.	150
Korkers (Nabisco)	1 piece	8
Corn & Sesame Chips (Nabisco)	1 piece	10
Creme Wafer Stick (Nabisco)	1 piece	47
Crown Pilot (Nabisco)	1 piece	75
Diggers (Nabisco)	1 piece	4
English Water Biscuit		
(Pepperidge Farm)	1 piece	17
Escort (Nabisco)	1 piece	21
French onion cracker (Nabisco)	1 piece	12
Goldfish (Pepperidge Farm):		
Thins	1 piece	10
Tiny	1 piece	3
Graham:		
(Dixie Belle) sugar-honey coated	1 piece	15

Food and Description	Measure or Quantity	Calories
Flavor Kist (Schulze and Burch) sugar-honey coated	1 piece	57
Honey Maid (Nabisco)	1 piece	30
Graham, chocolate or cocoa-covered:		
Fancy Dip (Nabisco)	1 piece	65
(Keebler)	1 piece	43
(Nabisco)	1 piece	57
Melba Toast (See MELBA TOAST)		
Milk lunch Biscuit (Keebler)	1 piece	27
Mucho Macho Nacho, Flavor Kist (Schulze and Burch)	1 oz.	121
Onion (Nabisco) French	1 piece	13
Oyster:		
(Dixie Belle)	1 piece	4
(Keebler) *Zesta*	1 piece	2
(Nabisco) *Dandy* or *Oysterettes*	1 piece	3
Pumpernickel Toast (Keebler)	1 piece	15
Ritz (Nabisco)	1 piece	17
Roman Meal Wafer, boxed	1 piece	11
Royal Lunch (Nabisco)	1 piece	55
Rusk, *Holland* (Nabisco)	1 piece	40
Rye toast (Keebler)	1 piece	16
RyKrisp:		
Natural	1 triple cracker	25
Seasoned or sesame	1 triple cracker	30
Saltine:		
(Dixie Belle) regular or unsalted	1 piece	12
Premium (Nabisco)	1 piece	12
Zesta (Keebler)	1 piece	13
Sea Toast (Keebler)	1 piece	60
Sesame:		
Butter flavored (Nabisco)	1 piece	17
Sesame Wheats! (Nabisco)	1 piece	17
Toast (Keebler)	1 piece	15
Shindigs (Keebler)	1 piece	6
Skittle Chips (Nabisco)	1 piece	14
Snackers (Ralston)	1 piece	17
Snackin' Crisp (Durkee) *D&C*	1 oz.	155
Snacks Sticks (Pepperidge Farm):		
Cheese	1 piece	17
Lightly salted, pumpernickel, rye & sesame	1 piece	16
Sociables (Nabisco)	1 piece	11
Table Wafer Cracker (Carr's) small	1 piece	15
Tortilla chips:		
(Bachman) nacho, taco flavor or toasted	1 oz.	140
Buenos (Nabisco)	1 piece	11

Food and Description	Measure or Quantity	Calories
Doritos, nacho or taco	1 oz.	140
(Nabisco) regular and nacho	1 piece	11
Town House Cracker (Keebler)	1 piece	16
Triscuit (Nabisco)	1 piece	20
Twigs (Nabisco)	1 piece	14
Uneeda Biscuit (Nabisco) unsalted	1 piece	22
Unsalted (Featherweight)	2 sections (½ cracker)	30
Waverley Wafer (Nabisco)	1 piece	18
Wheat (Pepperidge Farm) cracked or hearty	1 piece	28
Wheat Chips (Nabisco)	1 piece	4
Wheat Crisps (Keebler)	1 piece	13
Wheatmeal Biscuit (Carr's) small	1 piece	42
Wheat Snack (Dixie Belle)	1 piece	9
Wheatsworth (Nabisco)	1 piece	14
Wheat Thins (Nabisco)	1 piece	10
Wheat Toast (Keebler)	1 piece	15
Wheat wafer (Featherweight) unsalted	1 piece	13
CRACKER CRUMBS, graham (Nabisco)	⅛ of 9″ pie shell	70
CRACKER MEAL (Nabisco)	½ cup	220
CRANAPPLE JUICE (Ocean Spray) canned:		
Regular	6 fl. oz.	129
Dietetic	6 fl. oz.	32
CRANBERRY, fresh (Ocean Spray)	½ cup	26
CRANBERRY JUICE COCKTAIL:		
Canned (Ocean Spray):		
Regular	6 fl. oz.	106
Dietetic	6 fl. oz.	36
*Frozen (Welch's)	6 fl. oz.	100
CRANBERRY-ORANGE RELISH (Ocean Spray)	2 oz.	104
CRANBERRY-RASPBERRY SAUCE (Ocean Spray) jellied	2 oz.	89
CRANBERRY SAUCE:		
Home recipe, sweetened, unstrained	4 oz.	202
Canned (Ocean Spray):		
Jellied	2 oz.	88
Whole berry	2 oz.	89
CRANGRAPE (Ocean Spray)	6 fl. oz.	108
CRANTASTIC JUICE DRINK, canned (Ocean Spray)	6 fl. oz.	110
CRAZY COW, cereal (General Mills)	1 cup	110
CREAM:		
Half & half (Dairylea)	1 fl. oz.	40

Food and Description	Measure or Quantity	Calories
Light, table or coffee (Sealtest)		
16% fat	1 T.	26
Light, whipping, 30% fat (Sealtest)	1 T.	45
Heavy whipping (Dairylea)	1 fl. oz.	60
Sour (Dairylea)	1 fl. oz.	60
Sour, imitation (Pet)	1 T.	25
Substitute (See CREAM SUBSTITUTE)		
CREAM PUFFS:		
Home recipe, custard filling	3½" × 2" piece	303
Frozen (Rich's) chocolate	1⅓-oz. piece	146
CREAMSICLE (Popsicle Industries)	2½-fl.-oz. piece	80
CREAM SUBSTITUTE:		
Coffee Mate (Carnation)	1 tsp.	11
Dairy Light (Alba)	2.8-oz. envelope	10
N-Rich	3-gram packet	16
Perx	1 tsp.	8
(Pet)	1 tsp.	10
CREAM OF WHEAT, cereal:		
Regular	2½ T.	100
*Instant	1 T.	40
*Mix'n Eat:		
Regular	1 packet	100
Baked apple & cinnamon	1 packet	170
Banana & spice	1 packet	170
Maple & brown sugar	3¾ T.	170
Quick	1 T.	40
CREME DE BANANA LIQUEUR		
(Mr. Boston)	1 fl. oz.	93
CREME DE CACAO:		
(Hiram Walker)	1 fl. oz.	104
(Mr. Boston):		
Brown	1 fl. oz.	102
White	1 fl. oz.	93
CREME DE CASSIS (Mr. Boston)	1 fl. oz.	85
CREME DE MENTHE:		
(Bols)	1 fl. oz.	122
(Mr. Boston):		
Green	1 fl. oz.	109
White	1 fl. oz.	97
CREME DE NOYAUX (Mr. Boston)	1 fl. oz.	99
CREPE, frozen:		
(Mrs. Paul's):		
Crab	5½-oz. pkg.	248
Shrimp	5½-oz. pkg.	252
(Stouffer's):		
Chicken with mushroom sauce	8¼-oz. pkg.	390
Ham & asparagus	6¼-oz. pkg.	325

Food and Description	Measure or Quantity	Calories
Spinach with cheddar cheese sauce	9½-oz. pkg.	415
CRISP RICE CEREAL:		
(Featherweight) low sodium	1 cup	110
(Ralston Purina)	1 cup	110
CRISPY WHEATS'N RAISINS, cereal (General Mills)	¾ cup	110
CROUTON:		
(Arnold):		
Bavarian or English style	½ oz.	65
French, Italian or Mexican style	½ oz.	66
(Kellogg's) *Croutettes*	⅔ cup	70
(Pepperidge Farm):		
Cheddar & romano	.5 oz.	60
Cheese & garlic or seasoned	.5 oz.	70
C-3PO'S#, cereal (Kellogg's)	¾ cup	110
CUCUMBER:		
Eaten with skin	8-oz. cucumber	32
Pared,	7½″ × 2″ pared	29
Pared	3 slices (.9 oz.)	4
CUMIN SEED (French's)	1 tsp.	7
CUPCAKE:		
Regular (Hostess):		
Chocolate	1 cupcake	170
Orange	1 cupcake	150
Frozen (Sara Lee) yellow	1 cupcake	190
***CUPCAKE MIX** (Flako)	1 cupcake	150
CUP O'NOODLES (Nissin Foods):		
Beef	2½-oz. serving	343
Beef onion	2½-oz. serving	323
Chicken	2½-oz. serving	343
Chicken, twin pack	1.2-oz. serving	155
Shrimp	2½-oz. serving	336
CURAÇAO:		
(Bols)	1 fl. oz.	105
(Hiram Walker)	1 fl. oz.	96
CURRANT, DRIED (Del Monte)		
Zante	½ cup	204
CUSTARD:		
Chilled, *Swiss Miss*, chocolate or egg flavor	4-oz. container	150
*Mix, dietetic (Featherweight)	½ cup	80
C. W. POST, cereal:		
Plain	¼ cup	131
With raisins	¼ cup	128

D

Food and Description	Measure or Quantity	Calories
DAIRY QUEEN/BRAZIER:		
Banana split	13.5-oz. serving	540
Brownie Delight, hot fudge	9.4-oz. serving	600
Buster Bar	5¼-oz. piece	460
Chicken sandwich	7.8-oz. sandwich	67
Cone:		
Plain, any flavor, regular	5-oz. cone	240
Dipped, chocolate, regular	5½-oz. cone	340
Dilly Bar	3-oz. piece	210
Double Delight	9-oz. serving	490
DQ Sandwich	2.1-oz. sandwich	140
Fish sandwich:		
Plain	6-oz. sandwich	400
With cheese	6¼-oz. sandwich	440
Float	14-oz. serving	410
Freeze, vanilla	12-oz. serving	500
French fries:		
Regular	2½-oz. serving	200
Large	4-oz. serving	320
Frozen dessert	4-oz. serving	180
Hamburger:		
Plain:		
Single	5.2-oz. burger	360
Double	7.4-oz. burger	530
Triple	9.6-oz. burger	710
With cheese:		
Single	5.7-oz. burger	410
Double	8.4-oz. burger	650
Triple	10.63-oz. burger	820
Hot dog:		
Regular:		
Plain	3.5-oz. serving	280
With cheese	4-oz. serving	330
With chili	4½-oz. serving	320
Super:		
Plain	6.2-oz. serving	520
With cheese	6.9-oz. serving	580
With chili	7.7-oz. serving	570
Malt, chocolate:		
Small	10¼-oz. serving	520
Regular	14¾-oz. serving	760
Large	20¾-oz. serving	1060

Food and Description	Measure or Quantity	Calories
Mr. Misty:		
Plain:		
Small	8¼-oz. serving	190
Regular	11.64-oz. serving	250
Large	15½-oz. serving	340
Kiss	3.14-oz. serving	70
Float	14.5-oz. serving	390
Freeze	14.5-oz. serving	500
Onion rings	3-oz. serving	280
Parfait	10-oz. serving	430
Peanut Butter Parfait	10¾-oz. serving	750
Shake, chocolate:		
Small	10¼-oz. serving	490
Regular	14¾-oz. serving	710
Large	20¾-oz. serving	990
Strawberry shortcake	11-oz. serving	540
Sundae, chocolate:		
Small	3¾-oz. serving	190
Regular	6¼-oz. serving	310
Large	8¾-oz. serving	440
Tomato	½ oz.	4
DAIQUIRI COCKTAIL		
(Mr. Boston):		
Regular	3 fl. oz.	99
Strawberry	3 fl. oz.	111
DATE (Dromedary):		
Chopped	¼ cup	130
Pitted	5 dates	100
DE CHAUNAC WINE		
(Great Western) 12% alcohol	3 fl. oz.	71
DELI'S, frozen (Pepperidge Farm):		
Mexican style	4-oz. piece	280
Reuben in rye pastry	4-oz. piece	360
Turkey, ham & cheese	4-oz. piece	270
DESSERT CUPS (Hostess)	¾-oz. piece	62
DILL SEED (French's)	1 tsp.	9
DING DONG (Hostess)	1 cake	172
DINNER, FROZEN (See individual listings such as BEEF, CHICKEN, TURKEY, etc.)		
DIP:		
Avocado (Nalley's)	1 oz.	114
Barbecue (Nalley's)	1 oz.	114
Blue cheese:		
(Dean) tang	1 oz.	61
(Nalley's)	1 oz.	110
Clam (Nalley's)	1 oz.	101
Cucumber & onion (Breakstone)	1 oz.	50

Food and Description	Measure or Quantity	Calories
Enchilada, *Fritos*	1 oz.	37
Guacamole (Nalley's)	1 oz.	114
Jalapeno:		
Fritos	1 oz.	34
(Hain) natural	1 oz.	40
Onion bean (Hain) natural	1 oz.	41
DISTILLED LIQUOR, any brand:		
80 proof	1 fl. oz.	65
86 proof	1 fl. oz.	70
90 proof	1 fl. oz.	74
94 proof	1 fl. oz.	77
100 proof	1 fl. oz.	83
DONUTZ, cereal (General Mills)	1 cup	120
DOUGHNUT (See also *WINCHELL'S*):		
Regular (Hostess):		
Chocolate coated	1-oz. piece	130
Cinnamon	1-oz. piece	110
Donettes, powdered	1 piece	40
Old fashioned, plain	1.5-oz. piece	180
Powdered	1-oz. piece	110
Frozen (Morton):		
Regular:		
Boston creme	2-oz. piece	180
Chocolate iced	1.5-oz. piece	150
Jelly	1.8-oz. piece	180
Donut Holes	⅓ of 7¾-oz. pkg.	160
Morning Light, jelly	2.6-oz. piece	250
DRAMBUIE (Hiram Walker)	1 fl. oz.	110
DRUMSTICK, frozen:		
Ice Cream, in a cone:		
Topped with peanuts	1 piece	181
Topped with peanuts & cone bisque	1 piece	168
Ice Milk, in a cone:		
Topped with peanuts	1 piece	163
Topped with peanuts & cone bisque	1 piece	150
DUMPLINGS, canned, dietetic (Dia-Mel)	8-oz. serving	160

E

ECLAIR:

  Home recipe, with custard filling

    and chocolate icing

| | 4-oz. piece | 271 |

Description	Measure or Quantity	Calories
ECLAIR:		
Home recipe, with custard filling and chocolate icing	4-oz. piece	271
Frozen (Rich's) chocolate	1 piece	234
EEL, smoked, meat only	4 oz.	374
EGG, CHICKEN:		
Raw:		
White only	1 large egg	17
Yolk only	1 large egg	59
Boiled	1 large egg	81
Fried in butter	1 large egg	99
Omelet, mixed with milk & cooked in fat	1 large egg	107
Poached	1 large egg	78
Scrambled, mixed with milk & cooked in fat	1 large egg	111
EGG MIX (Durkee):		
Omelet:		
*With bacon	½ of pkg.	310
*Puffy	½ of pkg.	302
Scrambled:		
Plain	.8-oz. pkg.	124
With bacon	1.3-oz. pkg.	181
EGG NOG, dairy (Meadow Gold) 6% fat	½ cup	164
EGG NOG COCKTAIL (Mr. Boston) 15% alcohol	3 fl. oz.	180
EGGPLANT:		
Boiled, drained	4 oz.	22
Frozen:		
(Mrs. Paul's):		
Parmesan	5½-oz. serving	270
Sticks, breaded & fried	3½-oz. serving	262
(Weight Watchers) Parmesan	13-oz. pkg.	285
EGG ROLL, frozen (La Choy):		
Chicken	.4-oz. roll	30
Lobster	.4-oz. roll	27
Meat & shrimp	.2-oz. roll	17
Shrimp	3-oz. roll	160
EGG ROLL DINNER, frozen (Van de Kamp's) Cantonese	10½-oz. serving	550

Food and Description	Measure or Quantity	Calories
EGG, SCRAMBLED, FROZEN		
(Swanson) and sausage, with hashed brown potatoes, *TV Brand*	6½-oz. entree	430
EGG SUBSTITUTE:		
Egg Magic (Featherweight)	½ of envelope	60
Scramblers (Morningstar Farms)	1 egg substitute	35
Second Nature (Avoset)	3 T.	42
ENCHILADA OR ENCHILADA DINNER, frozen:		
Beef:		
(Banquet):		
Buffet Supper	2-lb. pkg.	1056
Dinner	12-oz-dinner	497
(Green Giant) Sonora style	12-oz. entree	700
(Hormel)	1 enchilada	140
(Morton)	11-oz. dinner	280
(Van de Kamp's):		
Dinner	12-oz. dinner	390
Entree, shredded	12-oz. entree	420
Cheese:		
(Banquet) Extra Helping	2-¼-oz. dinner	777
(Van de Kamp's)	12-oz. dinner	450
Chicken (Van de Kamp's)	7½-oz. pkg.	250
ENCHILADA SAUCE:		
Canned:		
(Del Monte) hot or mild	½ cup	45
Old El Paso, hot or mild	1 oz.	14
*Mix (Durkee)	½ cup	29
ENDIVE, CURLY OR ESCAROLE, cut	½ cup	7
EXPRESSO COFFEE LIQUEUR	1 fl. oz.	104

F

Food and Description	Measure or Quantity	Calories
FARINA:		
(Hi-O) dry, regular	1 T.	40
Malt-O-Meal, dry:		
Regular	1 oz.	96
Quick cooking	1 oz.	100
*(Pillsbury) made with milk and salt	⅔ cup	200
FAT, COOKING:		
Crisco:		
Regular	1 T.	110
Butter flavor	1 T.	126
Spry	1 T.	94
FENNEL SEED (French's)	1 tsp.	8
FETTUCINI ALFREDO, frozen (Stouffer's)	½ of 10-oz. pkg.	270
FIG:		
Small	1½" fig	30
Canned, regular pack (Del Monte) whole, solids & liq.	½ cup	100
Dried (Sun-Maid), Calimyrna	½ cup	250
FIG JUICE (Sunsweet)	6 fl. oz.	120
FIGURINES (Pillsbury) all flavors	1 bar	138
FILBERT:		
Shelled	1 oz.	180
(Fisher) oil dipped, salted	½ cup	360
FISH CAKE, frozen (Mrs. Paul's):		
Breaded & fried	2-oz. piece	105
Thins, breaded & fried	½ of 10-oz. pkg.	326
FISH & CHIPS, frozen:		
(Banquet) *Man-Pleaser*	14-oz. dinner	769
(Swanson):		
Hungry Man	15¾-oz. dinner	820
TV Brand	5-oz. entree	300
(Van de Kamp's) batter dipped, french fried	8-oz. pkg.	500
FISH DINNER, frozen:		
(Banquet)	8¾-oz. dinner	553
(Morton)	9-oz. dinner	260
(Mrs. Paul's) Parmesan	½ of 10-oz. pkg.	220
(Stouffer's) *Lean Cuisine,* Florentine	9-oz. pkg.	230
(Weight Watchers):		
Au gratin	9½-oz. meal	200
Oven fried	6¾-oz. meal	220

Food and Description	Measure or Quantity	Calories
FISH FILLET, frozen:		
(Mrs. Paul's):		
Batter fried, crunchy	2¼-oz. piece	155
Breaded & fried, light & natural	1 piece	290
Miniature, batter fried	3-oz. serving	181
(Van de Kamp's):		
Batter dipped, french fried	3-oz. piece	220
Country seasoned	2.4-oz. piece	180
FISH KABOBS, frozen:		
(Mrs. Paul's) light batter	⅓ pkg.	200
(Van de Kamp's) batter dipped, french fried	.4-oz. piece	26
FISH SEASONING (Featherweight)	¼ tsp.	<1
FISH STICK, frozen:		
(Mrs. Paul's):		
Batter fried	1 piece	69
Breaded & fried	1 piece	43
(Van de Kamp's) batter dipped, french fried	1-oz. piece	58
FIT'N FROSTY (Alba '77):		
Chocolate or marshmallow flavor	1 envelope	70
Strawberry	1 envelope	74
Vanilla	1 envelope	69
FIVE ALIVE (Snow Crop)	6 fl. oz.	85
FLOUNDER:		
Baked	4 oz.	229
Frozen:		
(Mrs. Paul's) fillets, breaded & fried	2-oz. piece	138
(Weight Watchers) with lemon-flavored bread crumbs	6½-oz. serving	134
FLOUR:		
(Aunt Jemima) self-rising	¼ cup	109
Ballard, self-rising	¼ cup	100
Bisquick (Betty Crocker)	¼ cup	120
(Elam's):		
Brown rice, whole grain	¼ cup	146
Buckwheat, pure	¼ cup	92
Pastry	1 oz.	102
Rye, whole grain	¼ cup	89
Soy	1 oz.	98
Gold Medal (Betty Crocker) all-purpose or high protein	¼ cup	100
La Pina	¼ cup	100
Pillsbury's Best:		
All-purpose or rye, medium	¼ cup	100
Sauce & gravy	2 T.	50
Self-rising	¼ cup	95

Food and Description	Measure or Quantity	Calories
Presto, self-rising	¼ cup	98
Wondra	¼ cup	100
FOOD STICKS (Pillsbury) chocolate	1 piece	45
FRANKEN*BERRY, cereal		
(General Mills)	1 cup	110
FRANKFURTER:		
(Eckrich):		
Beef, or meat	1.6-oz. frankfurter	150
Beef or meat, jumbo	2-oz. frankfurter	190
Meat	1.2-oz. frankfurter	120
(Hormel):		
Beef	1.6-oz. frankfurter	139
Range Brand, Wrangler, smoked	1 frankfurter	160
(Hygrade) beef, *Ball Park*	2-oz. frankfurter	169
(Louis Rich) turkey	1.5-oz. frankfurter	95
(Oscar Mayer):		
Beef	1.6-oz. frankfurter	145
Little Wiener	2″ frankfurter	31
Wiener	1.6-oz. frankfurter	145
Wiener, with cheese	1.6-oz. frankfurter	146
FRANKS-N-BLANKETS, frozen		
(Durkee)	1 piece	45
FRENCH TOAST, frozen:		
(Aunt Jemima):		
Regular	1 slice	85
Cinnamon swirl	1 slice	97
(Swanson) with sausage, *TV Brand*	4½-oz. pkg.	270
FRITTERS, FROZEN (Mrs. Paul's):		
Apple	2-oz. piece	125
Clam	1.9-oz. piece	131
Corn	2-oz. piece	73
Shrimp	½ of 7¾-oz. pkg.	242
FROOT LOOPS, cereal (Kellogg's)	1 cup	110
FROSTED RICE, cereal (Kellogg's)	1 cup	110
FROSTS (Libby's):		
Dry:		
Banana	.5 oz.	50
Orange, strawberry or pineapple	.5 oz.	60
Liquid:		
Banana	7 fl. oz.	120
Orange or strawberry	8 fl. oz.	120
FROZEN DESSERT, dietetic:		
Good Humor:		
Bar, vanilla with chocolate icing	2½-fl.-oz. bar	90
Cup, vanilla & chocolate	5-fl.-oz. cup	100
(SugarLo) all flavors	¼ pt.	135
FRUIT COCKTAIL:		
Canned, regular pack, solids & liq.:		
(Del Monte) regular or chunky	½ cup	94

Food and Description	Measure or Quantity	Calories
(Libby's)	½ cup	101
(Stokely-Van Camp)	½ cup	95
Canned, dietetic or low calorie, solids & liq.:		
(Del Monte) Lite	½ cup	58
(Diet Delight):		
Syrup pack	½ cup	50
Water pack	½ cup	40
(Featherweight):		
Juice pack	½ cup	50
Water pack	½ cup	40
(Libby's) water pack	½ cup	50
(S&W) *Nutradiet:*		
Juice pack	½ cup	50
Water pack	½ cup	40
***FRUIT COUNTRY** (Comstock):*		
Apple or blueberry	¼ of pkg.	160
Cherry	¼ of pkg.	180
FRUIT CUP (Del Monte):		
Mixed fruits	5-oz. container	110
Peaches, diced	5-oz. container	116
***FRUIT & FIBER CEREAL** (Post)*	½ cup	103
FRUIT JUICE, canned (Sun-Maid)	6 fl. oz.	100
FRUIT, MIXED:		
Canned (Del Monte) lite, chunky	½ cup	58
Frozen (Birds Eye) quick thaw	5-oz. serving	150
FRUIT PUNCH:		
Canned:		
Capri Sun	6¾ fl. oz.	102
(Hi-C)	6 fl. oz.	93
(Lincoln) party	6 fl. oz.	100
Chilled:		
Five Alive (Snow Crop)	6 fl. oz.	87
(Minute Maid)	6 fl. oz.	93
*Frozen, *Five Alive* (Snow Crop)	6 fl. oz.	87
*Mix (Hi-C)	6 fl. oz.	72
FRUIT ROLL, frozen (La Choy)	.5-oz. roll	38
***FRUIT ROLL-UPS** (Betty Crocker)*	1 piece	50
FRUIT SALAD:		
Canned, regular pack:		
(Del Monte) fruits for salad	½ cup	93
(Libby's)	½ cup	99
Canned, dietetic or low calorie:		
(Diet Delight)	½ cup	60
(Featherweight):		
Juice pack	½ cup	50
Water pack	½ cup	40

Food and Description	Measure or Quantity	Calories
(S&W) *Nutradiet:*		
Juice pack	½ cup	60
Water pack	½ cup	35
FRUIT SQUARES, frozen		
(Pepperidge Farm)	2½-oz. piece	230
FUDGSICLE (Popsicle Industries)	2½-fl.-oz. bar	100

G

Food and Description	Measure or Quantity	Calories
GARLIC:		
Flakes (Gilroy)	1 tsp.	5
Powder (French's)	1 tsp.	5
Spread (Lawry's)	1 T.	79
GEFILTE FISH, canned:		
(Mother's):		
Jellied, old world	4-oz. serving	70
Jellied, white fish & pike	4-oz. serving	60
In liquid broth	4-oz. serving	70
(Rokeach):		
Jellied, white fish & pike	4-oz. serving	50
Old Vienna	4-oz. serving	70
GELATIN, dry, *Carmel Kosher*	7-gram envelope	30
***GELATIN DESSERT MIX:**		
Regular:		
Carmel Kosher, all flavors	½ cup	80
(Jell-O) all flavors	½ cup	81
Dietetic:		
Carmel Kosher	½ cup	8
(D-Zerta) all flavors	½ cup	6
(Estee) all flavors	½ cup	40
(Featherweight) artificially		
sweetened or regular	½ cup	10
GELATIN, DRINKING (Knox)		
orange	1 envelope	70
GERMAN STYLE DINNER, frozen		
(Swanson) *TV Brand*	11¾-oz. dinner	370
GIN, SLOE:		
(Bols)	1 fl. oz.	85
(DeKuyper)	1 fl. oz.	70
(Mr. Boston)	1 fl. oz.	68
GINGER, powder (French's)	1 tsp.	6
***GINGERBREAD MIX:**		
(Betty Crocker)	⅑ of cake	210
(Dromedary)	2″ × 2″ square	100
(Pillsbury)	3″ square	190
GOLDEN GRAHAMS, cereal		
(General Mills)	¾ cup	110
GOOBER GRAPE (Smucker's)	1 oz.	125
GOOD HUMOR (See ICE CREAM)		

Food and Description	Measure or Quantity	Calories
GOOD N' PUDDIN		
(Popsicle Industries) all flavors	2⅓-fl.-oz. bar	170
GOOSE, roasted, meat & skin	4 oz.	500
GRAHAM CRAKOS, cereal		
(Kellogg's)	1 cup	110
GRANOLA BARS, *Nature Valley:*		
Almond, cinnamon or oats'n honey	1 bar	110
Coconut or peanut	1 bar	120
***GRANOLA BAR MIX,** chewy,		
Nature Valley, Bake-A-Bar	1 bar	100
GRANOLA CEREAL:		
Nature Valley:		
Cinnamon & raisin, fruit & nut or		
toasted oat	⅓ cup	130
Coconut & honey	⅓ cup	150
Sun Country:		
With almonds	½ cup	253
With raisins	½ cup	241
GRANOLA CLUSTERS,		
Nature Valley:		
Almond	1 piece	140
Caramel & raisin	1 piece	150
GRANOLA & FRUIT BAR,		
Nature Valley	1 bar	150
GRANOLA SNACK, *Nature Valley*	1 pouch	140
GRAPE:		
American, ripe (slipskin)	3½" × 3" bunch	43
Canned, dietetic (Featherweight)		
light, seedless, water pack	½ cup	60
GRAPE DRINK:		
Canned:		
Capri Sun	6¾-fl. oz.	104
(Hi-C)	6 fl. oz.	89
(Welchade)	6 fl. oz.	90
*Frozen (Welchade)	6 fl. oz.	90
*Mix (Hi-C)	6 fl. oz.	68
GRAPEFRUIT:		
Pink & red:		
Seeded type	½ med. grapefruit	46
Seedless type	½ med. grapefruit	49
White:		
Seeded type	½ med. grapefruit	44
Seedless type	½ med. grapefruit	46
Canned, regular pack (Del Monte)		
in syrup	½ cup	74
Canned, dietetic pack, solids & liq.:		
(Del Monte) sections ·	½ cup	45
(Diet Delight) sections	½ cup	45

Food and Description	Measure or Quantity	Calories
(Featherweight) sections, juice pack	½ cup	40
(S&W) *Nutradiet*	½ cup	40
GRAPEFRUIT DRINK, canned (Lincoln)	6 fl. oz.	104
GRAPEFRUIT JUICE:		
Fresh, pink, red or white	½ cup	46
Canned, sweetened:		
(Del Monte)	6 fl. oz.	89
(Texsun)	6 fl. oz.	77
Canned, unsweetened:		
(Del Monte)	6 fl. oz.	72
(Ocean Spray)	6 fl. oz.	64
(Texsun)	6 fl. oz.	77
Chilled (Minute Maid)	6 fl. oz.	75
GRAPEFRUIT JUICE COCKTAIL, canned (Ocean Spray) pink	6 fl. oz.	84
GRAPEFRUIT-ORANGE JUICE COCKTAIL, canned, *Musselman's*	6 fl. oz.	67
GRAPE JAM (Smucker's)	1 T.	53
GRAPE JELLY:		
Sweetened:		
(Smucker's)	1 T.	53
(Welch's)	1 T.	52
Dietetic:		
(Diet Delight)	1 T.	12
(Estee)	1 T.	18
(Featherweight) calorie reduced	1 T.	16
(Welch's)	1 T.	30
GRAPE JUICE:		
Canned, unsweetened:		
(Seneca Foods)	6 fl. oz.	118
(Welch's)	6 fl. oz.	120
*Frozen:		
(Minute Maid)	6 fl. oz.	99
(Welch's)	6 fl. oz.	100
GRAPE JUICE DRINK, chilled (Welch's)	6 fl. oz.	110
GRAPE NUTS, cereal (Post):		
Regular	¼ cup	108
Flakes	⅞ cup	108
Raisin	¼ cup	103
GRAVY, CANNED:		
Au jus (Franco-American)	2-oz. serving	10
Beef (Franco-American)	2-oz. serving	25
Brown:		
(Franco-American) with onion	2-oz. serving	25

Food and Description	Measure or Quantity	Calories
(Howard Johnson's)	½ cup	51
Ready Gravy	¼ cup	44
Chicken:		
(Franco-American):		
Regular	2-oz. serving	50
Giblet	2-oz. serving	26
Mushroom (Franco-American)	2-oz. serving	25
Turkey:		
(Franco-American)	2-oz. serving	30
(Howard Johnson's) giblet	½ cup	55
GRAVYMASTER	1 tsp.	11
GRAVY WITH MEAT OR TURKEY		
frozen:		
(Banquet):		
Buffet Supper, & sliced turkey	2-lb. pkg.	804
Cookin Bag, & sliced beef	4-oz. pkg.	136
(Morton) Family Meal, &		
sliced turkey	2-lb. pkg.	800
(Swanson) sliced beef with whipped		
potatoes, *TV Brand*	8-oz. entree	200
GRAVY MIX:		
Regular:		
Au jus:		
*(Durkee)	½ cup	15
*(French's) *Gravy Makins*	½ cup	16
Brown:		
*(Durkee) regular	½ cup	29
*(French's) *Gravy Makins*	½ cup	40
*(McCormick)	.85-oz. pkg.	82
*(Pillsbury)	½ cup	30
*(Spatini)	1 oz.	8
Chicken:		
*(Durkee) regular	½ cup	43
*(French's) *Gravy Makins*	½ cup	50
*(Pillsbury)	½ cup	50
Home style:		
*(Durkee)	½ cup	35
*(French's) *Gravy Makins*	½ cup	50
*(Pillsbury)	½ cup	30
Meatloaf (Durkee) *Roasting Bag*	1.5-oz. pkg.	129
Mushroom:		
*(Durkee)	½ cup	30
*(French's) *Gravy Makins*	½ cup	40
Onion:		
*(Durkee)	½ cup	42
*(French's) *Gravy Makins*	½ cup	50
*(McCormick)	.85-oz. pkg.	72

Food and Description	Measure or Quantity	Calories
Pork:		
*(Durkee)	½ cup	35
*(French's) *Gravy Makins*	½ cup	40
*Swiss Steak (Durkee)	½ cup	23
Turkey:		
*(Durkee)	½ cup	47
*(French's) *Gravy Makins*	½ cup	50
*Dietetic (Weight Watchers):		
Brown	½ cup	16
Brown, with mushroom	½ cup	24
Brown, with onion	½ cup	26
Chicken	½ cup	20
GREENS, MIXED, canned		
(Sunshine) solids & liq.	½ cup	20
GRENADINE (Garnier) no alcohol	1 fl. oz.	103
GUAVA	1 guava	48
GUAVA NECTAR (Libby's)	6 fl. oz.	70

H

Food and Description	Measure or Quantity	Calories
HADDOCK:		
Fried, breaded	4″ × 3″ × ½″ fillet	165
Frozen:		
(Banquet)	8¾-oz. dinner	419
(Mrs. Paul's) breaded & fried	2-oz. fillet	125
(Van de Kamp's) batter dipped, french fried	2-oz. piece	165
(Weight Watchers) with stuffing, 2-compartment	7-oz. pkg.	205
Smoked	4-oz. serving	117
HALIBUT:		
Broiled	4″ × 3″ × ½″ steak	214
Frozen (Van de Kamp's) batter dipped, french fried	½ of 8-oz. pkg.	270
HAM:		
Canned:		
(Hormel):		
Black Label (3- or 5-lb size)	4 oz.	140
Chunk	6¾-oz. serving	310
Patties	1 patty	180
(Oscar Mayer) *Jubilee,* extra lean, cooked	1-oz. serving	31
(Swift) *Premium*	1¾-oz. slice	111
Deviled:		
(Hormel)	1 T.	35
(Libby's)	1 T.	43
(Underwood)	1 T.	49
Packaged:		
(Eckrich):		
Loaf	1 oz.	70
Cooked or imported, danish	1.2-oz. slice	30
(Hormel):		
Black, or red peppered or frozen	1 slice	25
Chopped	1 slice	55
(Oscar Mayer):		
Chopped	1-oz. slice	64
Cooked, smoked	1-oz. slice	34
Jubilee, boneless:		
Sliced	8-oz. slice	264
Steak, 95% fat free	2-oz. steak	69

Food and Description	Measure or Quantity	Calories
HAMBURGER (See *McDONALD'S, BURGER KING, DAIRY QUEEN, WHITE CASTLE,* etc.)		
HAMBURGER MIX:		
Hamburger Helper (General Mills):		
Beef noodle, tomato or pizza dish	⅕ of pkg.	320
Cheeseburger Macaroni	⅕ of pkg.	360
Hash	⅕ of pkg.	300
Lasagna	⅕ of pkg.	330
Potatoes au gratin	⅕ of pkg.	320
Stew	⅕ of pkg.	290
Make a Better Burger (Lipton) mildly seasoned or onion	⅕ of pkg.	30
HAMBURGER SEASONING MIX:		
*(Durkee)	1 cup	663
(French's)	1-oz. pkg.	100
HAM & CHEESE:		
(Eckrich) loaf	1-oz. serving	60
(Hormel) loaf	1-oz. serving	65
HAM DINNER, frozen:		
(Banquet) American Favorites	10-oz. dinner	532
(Morton)	10-oz. dinner	440
HAM SALAD, canned (Carnation)	¼ of 7½-oz. can	110
HAM SALAD SPREAD (Oscar Mayer)	1 oz.	62
HAWAIIAN PUNCH:		
Canned:		
Cherry	6 fl. oz.	87
Grape	6 fl. oz.	93
*Mix, red punch	8 fl. oz.	100
HEADCHEESE (Oscar Mayer)	1-oz. serving	54
HERRING, canned (Vita):		
Cocktail, drained	8-oz. jar	342
In cream sauce	8-oz. jar	397
Tastee Bits, drained	8-oz. jar	361
HERRING, SMOKED, kippered	4-oz. serving	239
HICKORY NUT, shelled	1 oz.	191
HO-HO (Hostess)	1-oz. piece	120
HOMINY GRITS:		
Dry:		
(Albers)	1½ oz.	150
(Aunt Jemima)	3 T.	102
(Quaker):		
Regular	3 T.	101
Instant:		
Regular	.8-oz. packet	79
With imitation bacon or ham	1-oz. packet	101

Food and Description	Measure or Quantity	Calories
Cooked	1 cup	125
HONEY, strained	1 T.	61
HONEYCOMB, cereal (Post) regular	1⅓ cups	112
HONEYDEW	2″ × 7″ wedge	31
HONEY SMACKS, cereal (Kellogg's)	¾ cup	110
HORSERADISH:		
Raw, pared	1 oz.	25
Prepared (Gold's)	1 tsp.	3
HOSTESS O'S (Hostess)	2¾-oz. piece	277

I

Food and Description	Measure or Quantity	Calories
ICE CREAM (Listed by type, such as sandwich, or *Whammy*, or by flavor— see also FROZEN DESSERT):		
Bar (Good Humor) vanilla, chocolate coated	3-fl.-oz. piece	170
Butter pecan:		
(Breyer's)	¼ pt.	180
(Good Humor) bulk	4 fl. oz.	150
Cherry, black (Good Humor) bulk	4 fl. oz.	130
Chocolate:		
(Baskin-Robbins):		
Regular	1 scoop (2½ fl. oz.)	165
Fudge	1 scoop (2½ fl. oz.)	178
(Good Humor) bulk	4 fl. oz.	130
(Howard Johnson's)	½ cup	221
Chocolate chip (Good Humor)	4 fl. oz.	150
Chocolate chip cookie (Good Humor)	1 sandwich	480
Chocolate eclair (Good Humor) bar	3-fl.-oz piece	180
Coffee (Breyer's)	¼ pt.	140
Eskimo Pie, vanilla with chocolate coating	3-fl.-oz. bar	180
Eskimo, Thin Mint, with chocolate coating	2-fl.-oz. bar	140
Fudge royal (Good Humor) bulk	4 fl. oz.	120
Peach (Breyer's)	¼ pt.	130
Pralines 'N Cream (Baskin-Robbins)	1 scoop (2½ fl. oz.)	177
Sandwich (Good Humor)	2½-oz. piece	170
Strawberry:		
(Baskin-Robbins)	1 scoop (2½ fl. oz.)	141
(Good Humor) bulk	4 fl. oz.	120
(Howard Johnson's)	½ cup	187
Toasted almond bar (Good Humor)	3-fl.-oz. piece	190
Toffee fudge swirl (Good Humor) bulk	4 fl. oz.	130
Vanilla:		
(Baskin-Robbins) regular	1 scoop (2½ fl. oz.)	147
(Good Humor) bulk	4 fl. oz.	140
(Howard Johnson's)	½ cup	210
(Meadow Gold)	½ cup	140

Food and Description	Measure or Quantity	Calories
Vanilla-chocolate-strawberry (Good Humor)	4 fl. oz.	130
Vanilla fudge swirl (Good Humor) bulk	4 fl. oz.	140
Whammy (Good Humor):		
Assorted	1.6-oz. piece	90
Chip crunch bar	3-fl.-oz. piece	200
ICE CREAM CONE, cone only (Comet):		
Regular	1 piece	20
Rolled sugar	1 piece	40
ICE CREAM CUP, cup only (Comet)	1 cup	20
*ICE CREAM MIX (Salada) any flavor	1 cup	310
ICE MILK:		
Hardened	¼ pt.	100
Soft-serve	¼ pt.	133
(Dean) *Count Calorie*	¼ pt.	99
(Meadow Gold) vanilla, 4% fat	¼ pt.	95
ITALIAN DINNER, frozen (Banquet)	12-oz. dinner	597

J

Food and Description	Measure or Quantity	Calories
JELL-O FRUIT & CREAM BAR	1 bar	72
JELL-O GELATIN POPS:		
Cherry, grape or strawberry	1 pop	37
Raspberry	1 pop	34
JELL-O PUDDING POPS:		
Banana, butterscotch or vanilla	2-oz. piece	96
Chocolate or chocolate fudge	2-oz. piece	101
JELLY, sweetened (See also individual flavors)		
(Crosse & Blackwell) all flavors	1 T.	51
JERUSALEM ARTICHOKE, pared	4 oz.	75
JOHANNISBERG RIESLING WINE		
(Louis M. Martini)	3 fl. oz.	61

K

Food and Description	Measure or Quantity	Calories
KABOOM, cereal (General Mills)	1 cup	110
KALE:		
Boiled, leaves only	4 oz.	110
Canned (Sunshine) chopped, solids & liq.	½ cup	21
Frozen:		
(Birds Eye) chopped	⅓ of pkg.	32
(McKenzie) chopped	3⅓ oz.	25
(Southland) chopped	⅓ of 16-oz. pkg.	30
KARO SYRUP (See SYRUP)		
KEFIR (Alta-Dena Dairy):		
Plain	1 cup	180
Flavored	1 cup	190
KIDNEY:		
Beef, braised	4 oz.	286
Calf, raw	4 oz.	128
Lamb, raw	4 oz.	119
KIELBASA (Hormel) Kilbase	2-oz. serving	245
KING VITAMAN, cereal (Quaker)	1¼ cups	113
KIX, cereal	1½ cups	110
KNOCKWURST	1 oz.	79
*****KOOL-AID** (General Foods):		
Unsweetned (sugar to be added)	8 fl. oz.	98
Pre-sweetened:		
Regular, sugar sweetened:		
Apple or sunshine punch	8 fl. oz.	96
Cherry or grape	8 fl. oz.	89
Tropical punch	8 fl. oz.	99
Dietetic, sugar-free:		
Cherry or grape	8 fl. oz.	2
Sunshine punch	8 fl. oz.	4
KUMQUAT, flesh & skin	5 oz.	74

L

Food and Description	Measure or Quantity	Calories
LAMB:		
Leg:		
Roasted, lean & fat	3 oz.	237
Roasted, lean only	3 oz.	158
Loin, one 5-oz. chop (weighed with bone before cooking) will give you:		
Lean & fat	2.8 oz.	280
Lean only	2.3 oz.	122
Rib, one 5-oz. chop (weighed with bone before cooking) will give you:		
Lean & fat	2.9 oz.	334
Lean only	2 oz.	118
Shoulder:		
Roasted, lean & fat	3 oz.	287
Roasted, lean only	3. oz.	174
LASAGNA:		
Canned (Hormel) *Short Orders*	7½-oz. can	260
Frozen:		
(Green Giant):		
Bake:		
Regular, with meat sauce	12-oz. entree	490
Chicken	12-oz. entree	640
Boil 'N Bag	9½-oz. entree	290
(Stouffer's) *Lean Cuisine*	11-oz. meal	240
(Swanson):		
Hungry Man, with meat	17¾-oz. dinner	690
TV Brand	13-oz. dinner	420
(Van de Kamp's) creamy spinach	11-oz. meal	400
(Weight Watcher's) regular	12-oz. meal	360
LEEKS	4 oz.	59
LEMON:		
Whole	2⅛" lemon	22
Peeled	2⅛" lemon	20
LEMONADE:		
Canned:		
Capri Sun	6¾ fl. oz.	63
Country Time	6 fl. oz.	69
Chilled (Minute Maid) regular or pink	6 fl. oz.	79

Food and Description	Measure or Quantity	Calories
*Frozen:		
Country Time, regular or pink	6 fl. oz.	68
Minute Maid	6 fl. oz.	74
*Mix:		
Regular:		
Country Time, regular or pink	6 fl. oz.	68
(Hi-C)	6 fl. oz.	76
Kool-Aid, sweetened, regular or pink	6 fl. oz.	65
Lemon Tree (Lipton)	6 fl. oz.	68
Dietetic:		
Crystal Light	8 fl. oz.	4
Kool-Aid	6 fl. oz.	3
LEMON EXTRACT (Virginia Dare)	1 tsp.	21
LEMON JUICE:		
Canned, ReaLemon	1 T.	3
*Frozen (Minute Maid) unsweetened	1 fl. oz.	77
*LEMON-LIMEADE Drink, Crystal Light	8 fl. oz.	4
LEMON PEEL, candied	1 oz.	90
LENTIL, cooked, drained	½ cup	107
LETTUCE:		
Bibb or Boston	4" head	23
Cos or Romaine, shredded or broken into pieces	½ cup	4
Grand Rapids, Salad Bowl or Simpson	2 large leaves	9
Iceberg, New York or Great Lakes	¼ or 4¾" head	15
LIFE, cereal (Quaker) regular or cinnamon	⅔ cup	105
LIL' ANGELS (Hostess)	1-oz. piece	90
LIME, peeled	2" dia.	15
*LIMEADE, frozen (Minute Maid)	6 fl. oz.	75
LIME JUICE, ReaLime	1 T.	2
LINGUINI, frozen (Stouffer's) clam sauce	10½	285
LIVER:		
Beef:		
Fried	6½" × 2⅜" × ⅜"slice	195
Cooked (Swift)	3.2-oz. serving	141
Calf, fried	6½" × 2⅛" × ⅜"slice	222
Chicken, simmered	2" × 2" × ⅝" piece	41
LIVERWURST SPREAD (Hormel)	1-oz. serving	70
LOBSTER:		
Cooked, meat only	1 cup	138
Canned, meat only	4-oz. serving	108
Frozen, South African lobster tail 3 in 8-oz. pkg.	1 piece	87

Food and Description	Measure or Quantity	Calories
4 in 8-oz. pkg.	1 piece	65
5 in 8-oz. pkg.	1 piece	51
LOBSTER NEWBURG	1 cup	485
LOBSTER PASTE, canned	1-oz. serving	51
LOBSTER SALAD	4-oz. serving	125
LONG ISLAND TEA COCKTAIL (Mr. Boston) 12½% alcohol	3 fl. oz.	94
LOQUAT, fresh, flesh only	2 oz.	27
LUCKY CHARMS, cereal (General Mills)	1 cup	110
LUNCHEON MEAT (See also individual listings such as BOLOGNA, HAM, etc.):		
Banquet loaf (Eckrich)	¾-oz. slice	50
Bar-B-Que Loaf (Oscar Mayer) 90% fat free	1-oz. slice	49
Beef, jellied (Hormel) loaf	1.2-oz slice	45
Gourmet loaf (Eckrich)	1-oz. slice	35
Ham & cheese (See HAM & CHEESE)		
Ham roll sausage (Oscar Mayer)	1-oz. slice	43
Honey loaf:		
(Eckrich)	1-oz. slice	40
(Hormel)	1 slice	55
(Oscar Mayer) 95% fat free	1-oz. slice	37
Iowa brand (Hormel)	1 slice	45
Liver cheese (Oscar Mayer)	1.3-oz. slice	114
Liver loaf (Hormel)	1 slice	80
Macaroni-cheese loaf (Eckrich)	1-oz. slice	70
Meat Loaf	1-oz. serving	57
New England brand sliced sausage:		
(Eckrich)	1-oz. slice	35
(Oscar Mayer) 92% fat free	.8-oz slice	22
Old fashioned loaf (Oscar Mayer)	1-oz. slice	65
Olive loaf:		
(Eckrich)	1-oz. slice	80
(Hormel)	1-oz. slice	59
Peppered loaf:		
(Eckrich)	1-oz. slice	40
(Hormel)	1-oz. serving	72
(Oscar Mayer) 93% fat free	1-oz. slice	42
Pickle loaf:		
(Eckrich)	1-oz. slice	80
(Hormel)	1 slice	60
Pickel & pimiento (Oscar Mayer)	1-oz. slice	65
Spiced (Hormel)	1 slice	75

M

Food and Description	Measure or Quantity	Calories
MACADAMIA NUT		
(Royal Hawaiian)	1 oz.	197
MACARONI:		
Cooked:		
8-10 minutes, firm	1 cup	192
14-20 minutes, tender	1 cup	155
Canned (Franco-American):		
Beefy Mac	7½-oz. can	220
PizzOs	7½-oz. can	170
Frozen:		
(Banquet) *Buffet Supper*, & beef	2-lb. pkg.	1000
(Morton)	10-oz. dinner	260
(Swanson) *TV Brand*, & beef	12-oz. dinner	370
MACARONI & CHEESE:		
Canned:		
(Franco-American) regular or elbow	7⅜-oz. serving	170
(Hormel) *Short Orders*	7½-oz. can	170
Frozen:		
(Banquet):		
Buffet Supper	2-lb. pkg.	1344
Casserole	8-oz. pkg.	344
(Green Giant) *Boil 'N Bag*	9-oz.entree	290
(Morton)	8-oz. casserole	270
(Stouffer's)	6-oz. serving	260
(Swanson) *TV Brand*	12¼-oz. dinner	380
Mix:		
(Golden Grain) deluxe	¼ of 7¼-oz. pkg.	202
*(Prince)	¾ cup	268
MACARONI & CHEESE PIE,		
frozen (Swanson)	7-oz. pie	210
MACARONI SALAD, canned		
(Nalley's)	4-oz. serving	206
MACKEREL, Atlantic, broiled with fat	8½" × 2½" × ½"fillet	248
MALTED MILK MIX (Carnation):		
Chocolate	3 heaping tsps.	85
Natural	3 heaping tsps.	88
MALT LIQUOR, *Champale,* regular	12 fl. oz.	179
MALT-O-MEAL, cereal	1 T.	33

Food and Description	Measure or Quantity	Calories
MANDARIN ORANGE		
(See TANGERINE)		
MANGO, fresh	1 med. mango	88
MANGO NECTAR (Libby's)	6 fl. oz.	60
MANHATTAN COCKTAIL		
(Mr. Boston) 20% alcohol	3 fl. oz.	123
MAPLE SYRUP (See SYRUP, Maple)		
MARGARINE:		
Regular	1 pat (1″ × 1.3″ × 1″, 5 grams)	36
(Mazola)	1 T.	104
(Parkay) regular, soft or squeeze	1 T.	101
MARGARINE, IMITATION OR DIETETIC:		
(Parkay)	1 T.	55
(Weight Watchers)	1 T.	50
MARGARINE, WHIPPED		
(Blue Bonnet; Miracle; Parkay)	1 T.	67
MARGARITA COCKTAIL		
(Mr. Boston):		
Regular	3 fl. oz.	105
Strawberry	3 fl. oz.	138
MARINADE MIX:		
Chicken (Adolph's)	1-oz. packet	64
Meat:		
(Adolph's)	.8-oz. pkg.	38
(French's)	1-oz. pkg.	80
(Kikkoman)	1-oz. pkg.	64
MARJORAM (French's)	1 tsp.	4
MARMALADE:		
Sweetened:		
(Keiller)	1 T.	60
(Smucker's)	1 T.	53
Dietetic:		
(Dia-Mel; Louis Sherry)	1 T.	6
(Featherweight)	1 T.	16
(S&W) *Nutradiet*, red label	1 T.	12
MARSHMALLOW FLUFF	1 heaping tsp.	59
MARSHMALLOW KRISPIES, cereal		
(Kellogg's)	1¼ cups	140
MARTINI COCKTAIL (Mr. Boston):		
Gin, extra dry, 20% alcohol	3 fl. oz.	99
Vodka, 20% alcohol	3 fl. oz.	102
MASA HARINA (Quaker)	⅓ cup	137
MASA TRIGO (Quaker)	⅓ cup	149
MATZO (Horowitz-Margareten)		
regular	1 matzo	120

Food and Description	Measure or Quantity	Calories
MAYONNAISE:		
Real, *Hellmann's* (Best Foods)	1 T.	103
Imitation or dietetic:		
(Dia-Mel)	1 T.	106
(Diet Delight) *Mayo-Lite*	1 T.	24
(Featherweight) *Soyamaise*	1 T.	100
(Weight Watchers)	1 T.	40
***MAYPO*, cereal:**		
30-second	¼ cup	89
Vermont style	¼ cup	121
***McDONALD'S*:**		
Big Mac	1 hamburger	563
Cheeseburger	1 cheeseburger	307
Chicken McNuggets	1 serving	314
Chicken McNuggets Sauce:		
Barbecue	1.1-oz. serving	60
Honey	.5-oz. serving	50
Hot mustard or sweet & sour	1.1-oz. serving	63
Cookies:		
Chocolate chip	1 package	342
McDonaldland	1 package	308
Egg McMuffin	1 serving	327
Egg, scrambled	1 serving	180
English muffin, with butter	1 muffin	186
Filet-O-Fish	1 sandwich	432
Grapefruit juice	6 fl. oz.	80
Hamburger	1 hamburger	255
Hot cakes with butter & syrup	1 serving	500
Pie:		
Apple	1 pie	253
Cherry	1 pie	260
Potato:		
Fried	1 regular order	220
Hash browns	1 order	125
Quarter Pounder:		
Regular	1 hamburger	424
With cheese	1 hamburger	524
Sausage, pork	1 serving	206
Shake:		
Chocolate	1 serving	383
Strawberry	1 serving	362
Vanilla	1 serving	352
Sundae:		
Caramel	1 serving	328
Hot fudge	1 serving	310
Strawberry	1 serving	289

Food and Description	Measure or Quantity	Calories
MEATBALL DINNER or ENTREE, frozen:		
(Green Giant) sweet & sour	9.9-oz. entree	370
(Swanson) *TV Brand*	9¼-oz. entree	320
*MEATBALL SEASONING MIX (Durkee)		
Italian style	1 cup	619
MEATBALL STEW:		
Canned *Dinty Moore* (Hormel)	7½-oz. serving	245
Frozen (Stouffer's) *Lean Cuisine*	10-oz. serving	240
MEATBALLS, SWEDISH, frozen (Stouffer's) with noodles	11-oz. pkg.	475
MEAT LOAF DINNER, frozen:		
(Banquet):		
Buffet Supper	30-oz. pkg.	1510
Dinner, American Favorites	11-oz. dinner	437
(Morton) *Family Meal,* & tomato sauce	1-lb. pkg.	800
(Swanson) *TV Brand,* with tomato sauce & whipped potatoes	9-oz. entree	340
MEAT LOAF SEASONING MIX (Contadina)	3¾-oz. pkg.	360
MEAT, POTTED:		
(Hormel)	1 T.	30
(Libby's)	1-oz. serving	55
MEAT TENDERIZER:		
Regular (Adolph's; McCormick)	1 tsp.	2
Seasoned (McCormick)	1 tsp.	5
MELBA TOAST, salted (Old London):		
Garlic, onion or white rounds	1 piece	10
Pumpernickel, rye, wheat or white	1 piece	17
Sesame, flat	1 piece	18
MELON BALL, in syrup, frozen	½ cup	72
MERLOT WINE (Louis M. Martini) 12½% alcohol	3 fl. oz.	60
MEXICAN DINNER, frozen:		
(Morton)	11-oz. dinner	300
(Swanson) *TV Brand*	16-oz. dinner	590
(Van de Kamp's) combination	11-oz. dinner	430
MILK BREAK BARS (Pillsbury):		
Chocolate or chocolate mint	1 bar	230
Natural	1 bar	220
MILK, CONDENSED (Carnation)	1 T.	80
*MILK, DRY, non-fat, instant (Alba; Carnation, Pet; *Sanalac*)	1 cup	80

Food and Description	Measure or Quantity	Calories
MILK, EVAPORATED:		
Regular:		
(Carnation)	1 fl. oz.	42
(Pet)	1 fl. oz.	43
Filled (Pet)	½ cup	150
Low fat (Carnation)	1 fl. oz.	27
Skimmed, (Carnation; *Pet 99*)	1 fl. oz.	25
MILK, FRESH:		
Buttermilk (Friendship)	8 fl. oz.	120
Chocolate (Dairylea)	8 fl. oz.	180
Low fat, *Viva*, 2% fat	8 fl. oz.	130
Skim (Dairylea; Meadow Gold)	1 cup	90
Whole:		
(Dairylea)	1 cup	150
(Meadow Gold)	1 cup	120
MILK, GOAT, whole	1 cup	163
MILK, HUMAN	1 cup	163
MILNOT, dairy vegetable blend	1 fl. oz.	38
MINI-WHEATS, cereal (Kellogg's)		
frosted	1 biscuit	28
MINT LEAVES	½ oz.	4
MOLASSES:		
Barbados	1 T.	51
Blackstrap	1 T.	40
Dark (Brer Rabbit)	1 T.	33
Light	1 T.	48
Medium	1 T.	44
Unsulphured (Grandma's)	1 T.	60
MORTADELLA sausage	1 oz.	89
MOST, cereal (Kellogg's)	½ cup	100
MOUSSE, canned, dietetic		
(Featherweight) chocolate	½ cup	100
MUFFIN:		
Blueberry:		
(Morton) rounds	1.5-oz. muffin	110
(Pepperidge Farm)	1.9-oz. muffin	180
Bran (Arnold) *Bran'nola*	2.3-oz. muffin	160
Corn:		
(Morton)	1.7-oz. muffin	130
(Pepperidge Farm)	1.9-oz. muffin	180
(Thomas')	2-oz. muffin	184
English:		
(Arnold) extra crisp	2.3-oz. muffin	150
(Pepperidge Farm):		
Plain or wheat	2-oz. muffin	130
Cinnamon apple or sourdough	2-oz. muffin	140
Roman Meal	2.3-oz. muffin	150

Food and Description	Measure or Quantity	Calories
(Thomas's):		
Regular or frozen	2-oz. muffin	133
Raisin	2.2-oz. muffin	153
(Wonder)	2-oz. muffin	130
Orange-cranberry (Pepperidge Farm)	2.1-oz. muffin	190
Plain	1.4-oz. muffin	118
Sourdough (Wonder)	2-oz. muffin	130
MUFFIN MIX:		
Blueberry:		
*(Betty Crocker) wild	1 muffin	120
(Duncan Hines)	½2 of pkg.	99
Bran:		
(Duncan Hines)	½2 of pkg.	97
(Elam's) natural	1 T.	23
*Cherry (Betty Crocker)	½2 of pkg.	120
Corn:		
*(Betty Crocker)	1 muffin	160
*(Dromedary)	1 muffin	130
MULLIGAN STEW, canned, *Dinty Moore, Short Orders* (Hormel)	7½-oz. can	230
MUSCATEL WINE (Gallo)		
14% alcohol	3 fl. oz.	86
MUSHROOM:		
Raw, whole	½ lb.	62
Raw, trimmed, sliced	½ cup	10
Canned (Green Giant) solids & liq., whole or sliced:		
Regular	2-oz. serving	14
B in B	1½-oz. serving	18
MUSHROOM, CHINESE, dried	1 oz.	81
MUSSEL, in shell	1 lb.	153
MUSTARD:		
Powder (French's)	1 tsp.	9
Prepared:		
Brown (French's; Gulden's)	1 tsp.	5
Dijon, *Grey Poupon*	1 tsp.	6
Horseradish (Nalley's)	1 tsp.	5
Yellow (Gulden's)	1 tsp.	5
MUSTARD GREENS:		
Canned (Sunshine) solids & liq.	½ cup	22
Frozen:		
(Birds Eye)	⅓ of pkg.	25
(Southland)	⅓ of 16-oz. pkg.	20
MUSTARD SPINACH:		
Raw	1 lb.	100
Boiled, drained, no added salt	4-oz. serving	18

N

Food and Description	Measure or Quantity	Calories
NATURAL CEREAL:		
Heartland	¼ cup	138
(Quaker):		
Hot, whole wheat	⅓ cup	106
100%	¼ cup	138
100% with raisins & dates	¼ cup	134
NATURE SNACKS (Sun-Maid):		
Carob Crunch	1 oz.	143
Carob Peanut	1¼ oz.	190
Carob Raisin or Yogurt Raisin	1¼ oz.	160
Raisin Crunch or Rocky Road	1 oz.	126
Tahitian Treat or Yogurt Crunch	1 oz.	123
NECTARINE, flesh only	4 oz.	73
NOODLE:		
Dry (Pennsylvania Dutch Brand) broad	1 oz.	105
Cooked, 1½" strips	1 cup	200
NOODLES & BEEF:		
Canned (Hormel) *Short Orders*	7½-oz. can	230
Frozen (Banquet) *Buffet Supper*	2-lb. pkg.	754
NOODLES & CHICKEN:		
Canned (Hormel) *Dinty Moore, Short Orders*	7½-oz. can	210
Frozen (Swanson) *TV Brand*	10½-oz. dinner	270
NOODLE, CHOW MEIN (La Choy)	½ cup	150
NOODLE MIX:		
*(Betty Crocker):		
Fettucini Alfredo	¼ of pkg.	220
Romanoff	¼ of pkg.	230
Stroganoff	¼ of pkg.	240
Noodle Roni, parmesano	⅕ of 6-oz. pkg.	130
*(Lipton) *Egg Noodles & Sauce,* Beef, butter or chicken	¼ of pkg.	190
NOODLE, RICE (La Choy)	1 oz.	130
NOODLE ROMANOFF, frozen (Stouffer's)	⅓ of pkg.	170
NUT, MIXED:		
Dry roasted:		
(Flavor House)	1 oz.	172
(Planters)	1 oz.	160

Food and Description	Measure or Quantity	Calories
Oil roasted (Planters) with or without peanuts	1 oz.	180
NUTMEG (French's)	1 tsp.	11
NUTRI-GRAIN, cereal (Kellogg's):		
Corn	½ cup	110
Wheat	⅔ cup	110
Wheat & Raisin	⅔ cup	140
NUTRIMATO (Mott's)	6 fl. oz.	70

Food and Description	Measure or Quantity	Calories
OAT FLAKES, cereal (Post)	⅔ cup	107
OATMEAL:		
Dry:		
Regular:		
(Elam's) Scotch style	1 oz.	108
(H-O) old fashioned	1 T.	15
(Quaker) old fashioned	⅓ cup	109
(3-Minute Brand)	⅓ cup	110
Instant:		
(H-O):		
Regular, boxed	1 T.	15
With bran & spice	1½-oz. packet	157
With maple & brown sugar flavor	1½-oz. packet	160
(Quaker):		
Regular	1-oz. packet	105
Apple & cinnamon	1¼-oz. packet	134
Raisins & spice	1½-oz. packet	159
(3-Minute Brand)	½-oz. packet	162
Quick:		
(Harvest Brand)	⅓ cup	108
(H-O)	½ cup	129
(Ralston Purina)	⅓ cup	110
(3-Minute Brand)	⅓ cup	110
Cooked, regular	1 cup	132
OIL, SALAD OR COOKING:		
Crisco, Fleischman's; Mazola	1 T.	126
Mrs. Tucker's	1 T.	130
Sunlite: Wesson	1 T.	120
OKRA, frozen:		
(Birds Eye) whole, baby	⅓ of pkg.	36
(Seabrook Farms) cut	⅓ of pkg.	32
(Southland) cut	⅓ of 16-oz. pkg.	25
OLD FASHIONED COCKTAIL		
(Hiram Walker) 62 proof	3 fl. oz.	165
OLIVE:		
Green	4 med. or 3 extra large or 2 giant	19
Ripe, Mission	3 small or 2 large	18
OMELET, frozen (Swanson)		
TV Brand, Spanish style	7¾-oz. entree	240

Food and Description	Measure or Quantity	Calories
ONION:		
Raw	2½" onion	38
Boiled, pearl onion	½ cup	27
Canned (Durkee) *O & C:*		
Boiled	¼ of 16-oz. jar.	32
Creamed	¼ of 15½-oz. can	554
Dehydrated (Gilroy) flakes	1 tsp.	5
Frozen:		
(Birds Eye):		
Chopped	1 oz.	9
Creamed	⅓ of pkg.	106
Whole, small	⅓ of pkg.	44
(Green Giant) in cheese sauce	½ cup	90
(Mrs. Paul's) french-fried rings	½ of 5-oz. pkg.	167
(Southland) chopped	⅕ of 10-oz. pkg.	20
ONION BOUILLON:		
(Herb-Ox)	1 cube	10
MBT	1 packet	16
ONION, GREEN	1 small onion	4
ONION SALAD SEASONING		
(French's) instant	1 T.	15
ONION SALT (French's)	1 tsp.	6
ONION SOUP (See SOUP, Onion)		
ORANGE:		
Peeled	½ cup	62
Sections	4 oz.	58
ORANGE-APRICOT JUICE		
COCKTAIL, *Musselman's*	8 fl. oz.	100
ORANGE DRINK:		
Canned:		
Capri Sun	6¾-fl.-oz. can	103
(Hi-C)	8 fl. oz.	123
*Mix:		
Regular (Hi-C)	8 fl. oz.	91
Dietetic, *Crystal Light*	6 fl. oz.	4
ORANGE EXTRACT (Durkee)		
imitation	1 tsp.	15
ORANGE-GRAPEFRUIT JUICE:		
Canned (Libby's) unsweetened	6 fl. oz.	80
*Frozen (Minute Maid) unsweetened	6 fl. oz.	76
ORANGE JUICE:		
Canned:		
(Del Monte) unsweetened	6 fl. oz.	80
(Libby's) unsweetened	6 fl. oz.	90
(Texsun) sweetened	6 fl. oz.	83
Chilled (Minute Maid)	6 fl. oz.	83
*Frozen:		
(Birds Eye) Orange Plus	6 fl. oz.	95

Food and Description	Measure or Quantity	Calories
Bright & Early, imitation (Snow Crop)	6 fl. oz.	90
	6 fl. oz.	86
ORANGE PEEL, CANDIED	1 oz.	93
ORANGE-PINEAPPLE DRINK, canned (Lincoln)	8 fl. oz.	128
ORANGE-PINEAPPLE JUICE, canned (Texsun)	8 fl. oz.	89
OVALTINE, chocolate	¾ oz.	78
OVEN FRY (General Foods):		
Crispy crumb for pork	4.2-oz. evenlope	484
Crispy crumb for chicken	4.2-oz. envelope	460
Homestyle flour recipe	3.2-oz. envelope	304
OYSTER:		
Raw:		
Eastern	19-31 small or 13-19 med.	158
Pacific & Western	6-9 small or 4-6 med.	218
Canned (Bumble Bee) shelled, whole, solids & liq.	1 cup	218
Fried	4 oz.	271
OYSTER STEW, home recipe	½ cup	103

P

Food and Description	Measure or Quantity	Calories
PAC-MAN CEREAL (General Mills)	1 cup	110
***PANCAKE BATTER FROZEN** (Aunt Jemima):		
Plain	4" pancake	70
Blueberry or buttermilk	4" pancake	68
PANCAKE & SAUSAGE, frozen (Swanson)	6-oz. entree	440
***PANCAKE & WAFFLE MIX:**		
Plain:		
(Aunt Jemima) Original	4" pancake	73
(Log Cabin) Complete	4" pancake	58
(Pillsbury) *Hungry Jack:*		
Complete, bulk	4" pancake	63
Extra Lights	4" pancake	70
Golden Blend, complete	4" pancake	80
Panshakes	4" pancake	83
Blueberry (Pillsbury) *Hungry Jack*	4" pancake	107
Buckwheat (Aunt Jemima)	4" pancake	67
Buttermilk:		
(Aunt Jemima) regular	4" pancake	100
(Betty Crocker) complete	4" pancake	70
(Pillsbury) *Hungry Jack,* complete	4" pancake	63
Whole wheat (Aunt Jemima)	4" pancake	83
Dietetic:		
(Dia-mel)	3" pancake	33
(Featherweight)	4" pancake	43
PANCAKE & WAFFLE SYRUP (See SYRUP, Pancake & Waffle)		
PAPAYA, fresh:		
Cubed	½ cup	36
Juice	4 oz.	78
PAPRIKA (French's)	1 tsp.	7
PARSLEY:		
Fresh, chopped	1 T.	2
Dried (French's)	1 tsp.	4
PASSION FRUIT, giant, whole	1 lb.	53
PASTINAS, egg	1 oz.	109
PASTRAMI (Eckrich) sliced	1-oz. serving	40
PASTRY SHEET, PUFF, frozen (Pepperidge Farm)	1 sheet	510

Food and Description	Measure or Quantity	Calories
PÂTÉ:		
De foie gras	1 T.	69
Liver:		
(Hormel)	1 T.	35
(Sell's)	1 T.	93
PDQ:		
Chocolate	1 T.	66
Strawberry	1 T.	60
PEA, green:		
Boiled	½ cup	58
Canned, regular pack, solids & liq.:		
(Del Monte) seasoned or sweet, regular size	½ cup	60
(Green Giant):		
Early with onions, sweet or sweet with onions	¼ of 17-oz. can	60
Sweet, mini	¼ of 17-oz. can	64
(Libby's) sweet	½ cup	66
Canned, dietetic pack, solids & liq.:		
(Del Monte) No Salt Added, sweet	½ cup	60
(Diet Delight)	½ cup	50
(Featherweight) sweet	½ cup	70
(S&W) *Nutradiet*	½ cup	40
Frozen:		
(Birds Eye):		
Regular	⅓ of pkg.	78
In butter sauce	⅓ of pkg.	85
In cream sauce	⅓ of pkg.	84
(Green Giant):		
In cream sauce	½ cup	100
Early June or sweet, polybag	½ cup	60
Early & sweet in butter sauce	½ cup	90
Sweet, *Harvest Fresh*	½ cup	80
PEA & CARROT:		
Canned, regular pack, solids & liq.:		
(Del Monte)	½ cup	50
(Libby's)	½ cup	56
Canned, dietetic pack, solids & liq.:		
(Diet Delight)	½ cup	40
(S&W) *Nutradiet*	½ cup	35
Frozen:		
(Birds Eye)	⅓ of pkg.	61
(McKenzie)	3.3-oz. serving	60
PEA, CROWDER, frozen		
(Southland)	⅓ of 16-oz. pkg.	120

Food and Description	Measure or Quantity	Calories
PEA POD:		
Boiled, drained solids	4 oz.	49
Frozen (La Choy)	6-oz. pkg.	70
PEACH:		
Fresh, with thin skin	2″ peach	38
Fresh, slices	½ cup	32
Canned, regular pack, solids & liq.:		
(Del Monte) Cling:		
Halves or slices	½ cup	80
Spiced	3½ oz.	80
(Libby's) heavy syrup:		
Halves	½ cup	105
Sliced	½ cup	102
Canned, dietetic pack, solids & liq.:		
(Del Monte) Lite, Cling	½ cup	50
(Diet Delight) Cling:		
Juice pack	½ cup	50
Water Pack	½ cup	30
(Featherweight):		
Cling or Freestone, juice pack	½ cup	50
Cling, water pack	½ cup	30
(S&W) *Nutradiet,* Cling:		
Juice pack	½ cup	60
Water pack	½ cup	30
Frozen (Birds Eye)	5-oz. pkg.	141
PEACH BUTTER (Smucker's)	1 T.	45
PEACH DRINK, canned (Hi-C):		
Canned	6. fl.oz.	90
*Mix	6 fl. oz.	72
PEACH LIQUEUR (DeKuyper)	1 fl. oz.	82
PEACH NECTAR, canned (Libby's)	6 fl. oz.	90
PEACH PRESERVE OR JAM:		
Sweetened (Smucker's)	1 T.	53
Dietetic (Dia-Mel)	1 T.	6
PEANUT:		
Dry roasted:		
(Fisher)	1 oz.	163
(Planters)	1 oz.	160
Oil roasted (Planters)	1 oz.	179
PEANUT BUTTER:		
Regular:		
(Elam's) natural	1 T.	109
(Jif) creamy	1 T.	93
(Peter Pan):		
Crunchy	1 T.	101
Smooth	1 T.	94

Food and Description	Measure or Quantity	Calories
(Skippy):		
Creamy or super chunk	1 T.	108
Creamy, old fashioned	1 T.	107
Dietetic:		
(Featherweight) low sodium	1 T.	90
(Peter Pan) low sodium	1 T.	106
(S&W) *Nutradiet*, low sodium	1 T.	93
PEANUT BUTTER BAKING CHIPS (Reese's)	3 T. (1 oz.)	151
PEAR:		
Whole	3" × 2½" pear	101
Canned, regular pack, solids & liq.:		
(Del Monte) Bartlett	½ cup	80
(Libby's)	½ cup	102
Canned, dietetic pack, solids & liq.:		
(Del Monte) Lite	½ cup	50
(Featherweight) Bartlett:		
Juice pack	½ cup	60
Water pack	½ cup	40
(Libby's) water pack	½ cup	60
Dried (Sun-Maid)	½ cup	260
PEAR NECTAR, canned (Libby's)	6 fl. oz.	100
PEAR-PASSION FRUIT NECTAR, canned (Libby's)	6 fl. oz.	60
PEBBLES, cereal:		
Cocoa	⅞ cup	117
Fruity	⅞ cup	116
PECAN:		
Halves	6-7 pieces	48
Roasted, dry:		
(Fisher) salted	1 oz.	220
(Planters)	1 oz.	190
PECTIN, FRUIT:		
Certo	6-oz. pkg.	19
Sure-Jell	1¾-oz. pkg.	170
PEPPER:		
Black (French's)	1 tsp.	9
Lemon (Durkee)	1 tsp.	1
Seasoned (French's)	1 tsp.	8
PEPPER, CHILI, canned:		
(Del Monte):		
Green, whole	½ cup	20
Jalapeno or chili, whole	½ cup	30
Old El Paso, green, chopped or whole	1 oz.	7
(Ortega):		
Diced, strips or whole	1 oz.	6
Jalapeno, diced or whole	1 oz.	9

Food and Description	Measure or Quantity	Calories
PEPPERMINT EXTRACT (Durkee) imitation	1 tsp.	15
PEPPERONI:		
(Eckrich)	1-oz. serving	135
(Hormel) regular or Rosa Grande	1-oz. serving	140
PEPPER & ONION, frozen (Southland):		
Diced	2-oz. serving	15
Red & green	2-oz. serving	20
PEPPER STEAK, frozen (Stouffer's)	5¼-oz. serving	354
PEPPER, STUFFED:		
Home recipe	2¾″ × 2½″ pepper with 1⅛ cups stuffing	314
Frozen:		
(Green Giant) green, baked	7-oz. serving	200
(Stouffer's) green	7¾-oz. serving	225
(Weight Watchers) with veal stuffing	11¾-oz. meal	240
PEPPER, SWEET:		
Raw:		
Green:		
Whole	1 lb.	82
Without stem & seeds	1 med. pepper (2.6 oz.)	13
Red:		
Whole	1 lb.	112
Without stem & seeds	1 med. pepper (2.2 oz.)	19
Boiled, green, without salt, drained	1 med. pepper (2.6 oz.)	13
Frozen:		
(McKenzie)	1-oz. serving	6
(Southland):		
Green	2-oz. serving	10
Red & green	2-oz. serving	15
PERCH, OCEAN:		
Atlantic, raw:		
Whole	1 lb.	124
Meat only	4 oz.	108
Pacific, raw, whole	1 lb.	116
Frozen:		
(Banquet)	8¾-oz. dinner	434
(Mrs. Paul's) fillet, breaded & fried	2-oz. piece	145
(Van de Kamp's) batter dipped, french fried	2-oz. piece	145
PERNOD (Julius Wile)	1 fl. oz.	79

Food and Description	Measure or Quantity	Calories
PERSIMMON:		
Japanese or Kaki, fresh:		
With seeds	4.4-oz. piece	79
Seedless	4.4-oz. piece	81
Native, fresh, flesh only	4-oz. serving	144
PHEASANT, raw, meat only	4-oz. serving	184
PICKLE:		
Cucumber, fresh or bread & butter:		
(Fannings)	1.2-oz. serving	17
(Featherweight) low sodium	1-oz. pickle	12
(Nalley's) chips	1-oz. serving	27
Dill:		
(Featherweight) low sodium, whole	1-oz. serving	4
(Smucker's):		
Hamburger, sliced	1 slice	Tr.
Polish, whole	3½″ pickle	8
Spears	3½″ spear	6
Hamburger (Nalley's) chips	1-oz. serving	3
Kosher dill:		
(Claussen) halves or whole	2-oz. serving	7
(Featherweight) low sodium	1-oz. serving	4
(Smucker's):		
Baby	2¾-oz. long pickle	4
Slices	1 slice	Tr.
Whole	2½″ long pickle	8
Sweet:		
(Nalley's) *Nubbins*	1-oz. serving	28
(Smucker's):		
Candied mix	1 piece	14
Gherkins	2″ long pickle	15
Whole	2½″ long pickle	18
Sweet & sour (Claussen) slices	1 slice	3
PIE:		
Regular, non-frozen:		
Apple:		
Home recipe, two crust	⅙ of 9″ pie	404
(Hostess)	4½-oz. pie	390
Banana, home recipe, cream or custard	⅙ of 9″ pie	336
Berry (Hostess)	4½-oz. pie	404
Blackberry, home recipe, two-crust	⅙ of 9″ pie	384
Blueberry:		
Home recipe, two-crust	⅙ of 9″ pie	382
(Hostess)	4½-oz. pie	394
Boston cream, home recipe	1/12 of 8″ pie	208

Food and Description	Measure or Quantity	Calories
Buterscotch, home recipe, one-crust	1/6 of 9" Pie	406
Cherry:		
Home recipe, two-crust	1/6 of 9" pie	412
(Hostess)	4½-oz. pie	390
Chocolate chiffon, home recipe	1/6 of 9" pie	459
Chocolate meringue, home recipe	1/6 of 9"pie	353
Coconut custard, home recipe	1/6 of 9"pie	357
Lemon (Hostess)	4½-oz. pie	400
Mince, home recipe, two-crust	1/6 of 9" pie	428
Peach (Hostess)	4½-oz. pie	400
Pumpkin, home recipe, one-crust	1/6 of 9" pie	321
Raisin, home recipe, two-crust	1/6 of 9" pie	427
Strawberry (Hostess)	4½-oz. pie	340
Frozen:		
Apple:		
(Banquet) family size	1/5 of 20-oz. pie	263
(Morton):		
Regular	1/6 of 24-oz. pie	296
Great Little Desserts, regular	8-oz. pie	590
(Sara Lee) regular	1/6 of 31-oz. pie	376
Banana cream:		
(Banquet)	1/6 of 14-oz. pie	172
(Morton) regular	1/6 of 16-oz. pie	174
Blackberry (Banquet)	1/6 of 20-oz. pie	268
Blueberry:		
(Banquet)	1/6 of 20-oz. pie	266
(Morton) *Great Little Desserts*	8-oz. pie	580
(Sara Lee)	1/5 of 31-oz. pie	449
Cherry:		
(Banquet) regular	8-oz. pie	575
(Morton) regular	1/6 of 24-oz. pie	300
(Sara Lee)	1/6 of 31-oz. pie	397
Chocolate (Morton)	1/6 of 14-oz. pie	180
Chocolate cream:		
(Banquet)	1/6 of 14-oz. pie	177
(Morton) *Great Little* Desserts	3½-oz. pie	270
Coconut cream (Banquet)	1/6 of 14-oz. pie	179
Coconut custard (Morton) *Great Little Desserts*	6½-oz. pie	370
Lemon cream:		
(Banquet)	1/6 of 14-oz. pie	168
(Morton) *Great Little Desserts*	3½-oz. pie	250
Mince:		
(Banquet)	1/6 of 20-oz. pie	258
(Morton)	1/6 of 24-oz. pie	310
Peach (Sara Lee)	1/6 of 31-oz. pie	458

Food and Description	Measure or Quantity	Calories
Pumpkin:		
(Banquet)	⅙ of 20-oz. pie	197
(Morton) regular	⅙ of 24-oz. pie	230
(Sara Lee)	⅛ of 45-oz. pie	354
Strawberry cream (Banquet)	⅙ of 14-oz. pie	168
PIECRUST:		
Home recipe, 9″ pie	1 crust	900
Frozen (Banquet) 9″ shell:		
Regular	1 crust	614
Deep Dish	1 crust	751
Refrigerated (Pillsbury)	2 crusts	1920
*PIECRUST MIX:		
(Betty Crocker):		
Regular	¹⁄₁₆ of pkg.	120
Stick	⅛ of stick	120
(Flako)	⅙ of 9″ pie shell	245
(Pillsbury) mix or stick	⅙ of 2-crust pie	270
PIE FILLING (See also PUDDING OR PIE FILLING):		
Apple (Comstock)	⅙ of 21-oz. can	110
Apple rings or slices (See APPLE, canned)		
Apricot (Comstock)	⅙ of 21-oz. can	110
Banana cream (Comstock)	⅙ of 21-oz. can	110
Blueberry (Comstock)	⅙ of 21-oz. can	120
Coconut cream (Comstock)	⅙ of 21-oz. can	120
Coconut custard, home recipe, made with egg yolk & milk	5 oz. (inc. crust)	288
Lemon (Comstock)	⅙ of 21-oz. can	160
Mincemeat (Comstock)	½ of 21-oz. can	170
Pumpkin (Libby's) (See also PUMPKIN, canned)	1 cup	210
Raisin (Comstock)	⅙ of 21-oz. can	140
*PIE MIX (Betty Crocker)		
Boston cream	⅛ of pie	260
PIEROGIES, frozen (Mrs. Paul's)		
potato & cheese	1 pierogi	93
PIGS FEET, pickled	4-oz. serving	226
PIMIENTO, canned:		
(Dromedary)	1-oz. serving	10
(Ortega)	¼ cup	6
(Sunshine) diced or sliced	1 T.	4
PIÑA COLADA (Mr. Boston)		
12½% alcohol	3 fl. oz.	240
PINEAPPLE:		
Fresh, chunks	½ cup	52
Canned, regular pack, solids & liq.:		
(Del Monte) slices, syrup pack	½ cup	90

95

Food and Description	Measure or Quantity	Calories
(Dole):		
Juice pack, chunk, crushed or sliced	½ cup	70
Heavy syrup, chunk, crushed or sliced	½ cup	95
Canned, unsweetened or dietetic, solids & liq.:		
(Diet Delight) juice pack	½ cup	70
(Libby's) Lite	½ cup	60
(S&W) *Nutradiet*	1 slice	30
PINEAPPLE, CANDIED	1-oz. serving	90
PINEAPPLE FLAVORING (Durkee) imitation	1 tsp.	6
PINEAPPLE & GRAPEFRUIT JUICE DRINK, canned:		
(Del Monte) regular or pink	6 fl. oz.	90
(Dole) pink	6 fl. oz.	101
(Texsun)	6 fl. oz.	91
Canned:		
(Del Monte)	6 fl. oz.	100
(Dole)	6 fl. oz.	103
(Texsun)	6 fl. oz.	97
*Frozen (Minute Maid)	6 fl. oz.	92
PINEAPPLE-ORANGE DRINK, canned (Hi-C)	6 fl. oz.	94
PINEAPPLE-ORANGE JUICE:		
Canned (Del Monte)	6 fl. oz.	90
*Frozen (Minute Maid)	6 fl. oz.	94
PINEAPPLE PRESERVE OR JAM, sweetened (Smucker's)	1 T.	53
PINE NUT, pignolias, shelled	1 oz.	156
PINOT CHARDONNAY WINE (Paul Masson) 12% alcohol	3 fl. oz.	71
PISTACHIO NUT:		
In shell	½ cup	197
Shelled	¼ cup	184
(Fisher) shelled, roasted, salted	1 oz.	174
PIZZA PIE:		
Regular, non-frozen:		
Home recipe	⅛ of 14″ pie	177
(Pizza Hut):		
Cheese	½ of 10″ pie	436
Pepperoni	½ of 10″ pie	459
Frozen:		
Canadian style bacon (Celeste)	8-oz. pie	483
Cheese:		
(Celeste)	¼ of 19-oz. pie	309

Food and Description	Measure or Quantity	Calories
(Stouffer's) French Bread	½ of 10⅜-oz. pkg.	330
(Weight Watchers)	6-oz. pie	350
Combination:		
(Celeste) Chicago style	¼ of 24-oz. pie	360
(La Pizzeria)	½ of 13½-oz. pie	420
(Van de Kamp's) thick crust	¼ of 24½-oz. pie	310
(Weight Watchers)	7¼-oz. pie	322
Deluxe:		
(Celeste)	½ of 9-oz. pie	281
(Stouffer's) French Bread	½ of 12⅜-oz. pkg.	400
Hamburger (Stouffer's) French Bread	½ of 12¼-oz. pkg.	400
Mexican style (Van de Kamp's)	½ of 11-oz. pkg.	420
Mushroom (Stouffer's) French Bread	½ of 12-oz. pkg.	340
Pepperoni:		
(Celeste)	¼ of 20-oz. pie	347
(Stouffer's) French Bread	½ of 11¼-oz. pkg.	410
(Van de Kamp's) thick crust	¼ of 22-oz. pie	370
Sausage:		
(Celeste)	½ of 8-oz. pie	262
(Stouffer's) French Bread	½ of 12-oz. pkg.	420
(Weight Watchers) veal	6¾-oz. pie	350
Sausage & mushroom:		
(Celeste)	¼ of 24-oz. pie	365
(Stouffer's) French Bread	½ of 12½-oz. pkg.	395
Sicilian style (Celeste) deluxe	¼ of 26-oz. pie	408
Supreme (Celeste) without meat	½ of 8-oz. pie	217
Vegetable (Weight Watchers)	7¼-oz. pie	350
*Mix (Ragu) Pizza Quick	¼ of pie	300
PIZZA SAUCE:		
(Contadina):		
Regular or with cheese	½ cup	80
With pepperoni	½ cup	90
(Ragu):		
Regular	2 oz.	35
Pizza Quick	2 oz.	45
PLUM:		
Fresh, Japanese & hybrid	2" plum	27
Fresh, prune-type, halves	½ cup	60
Canned, regular pack (Stokely-Van Camp)	½ cup	120
Canned, unsweetened, purple, solids & liq.:		
(Diet Delight) juice pack	½ cup	70
(Featherweight) water pack	½ cup	40
(S&W) *Nutradiet*, juice pack	½ cup	80

Food and Description	Measure or Quantity	Calories
PLUM PRESERVE OR JAM,		
sweetened (Smucker's)	1 T.	53
PLUM PUDDING (Richardson &		
Robbins)	2" wedge	270
POLYNESIAN-STYLE DINNER,		
frozen (Swanson) *TV Brand*	12-oz. dinner	350
POMEGRANATE, whole	1 lb.	160
PONDEROSA RESTAURANT:		
A-1 Sauce	1 tsp.	4
Beef, chopped (patty only):		
Regular	3½ oz.	209
Double Deluxe	5.9 oz.	362
Junior (*Square Shooter*)	1.6 oz.	98
Steakhouse Deluxe	2.96 oz.	181
Beverages:		
Coca-Cola	8 fl. oz.	96
Coffee	6 fl. oz.	2
Dr. Pepper	8 fl. oz.	96
Milk, chocolate	8 fl. oz.	208
Orange drink	8 fl. oz.	110
Root beer	8 fl. oz.	104
Sprite	8 fl. oz.	95
Tab	8 fl. oz.	1
Bun:		
Regular	2.4-oz. bun	190
Hot dog	1 bun	108
Junior	1.4-oz. bun	118
Steakhouse deluxe	2.4-oz. bun	190
Chicken strips:		
Adult portion	2¾ oz.	282
Child	1.4 oz.	141
Cocktail sauce	1½ oz.	57
Filet Mignon	3.8 oz. (edible portion)	57
Filet of sole, fish only (See also Bun)	3-oz. piece	125
Fish, baked	4.9-oz. serving	268
Gelatin dessert	½ cup	97
Gravy, au jus	1 oz.	3
Ham & cheese:		
Bun (see Bun)		
Cheese, Swiss	2 slices (.8 oz.)	76
Ham	2½ oz.	184
Hot dog, child's, meat only (see also Bun)	1.6-oz. hot dog	140
Margarine:		
Pat	1 tsp.	36
On potato, as served	½ oz.	100

Food and Description	Measure or Quantity	Calories
Mustard sauce, sweet & sour	1 oz.	50
New York strip steak	6.1 oz. (edible portion)	362
Onion, chopped	1 T.	4
Pickle, dill	3 slices (.7 oz.)	2
Potato:		
Baked	7.2-oz. potato	145
French fries	3-oz. serving	230
Prime ribs:		
Regular	4.2 oz. (edible portion)	286
Imperial	8.4 oz. (edible portion)	572
King	6 oz. edible portion	409
Pudding, chocolate	4½ oz.	213
Ribeye	3.2 oz. (edible portion)	197
Ribeye & Shrimp:		
Ribeye	3.2 oz.	197
Shrimp	2.2 oz.	139
Roll, kaiser	2.2-oz. roll	184
Salad bar:		
Bean sprouts	1 oz.	13
Beets	1 oz.	5
Broccoli	1 oz.	9
Cabbage, red	1 oz.	9
Carrots	1 oz.	12
Cauliflower	1 oz.	8
Celery	1 oz.	4
Chickpeas (Garbanzos)	1 oz.	102
Cucumber	1 oz.	4
Mushrooms	1 oz.	8
Onion, white	1 oz.	11
Pepper, green	1 T.	6
Radish	1 oz.	5
Tomato	1 oz.	6
Salad dressing:		
Blue cheese	1 oz.	129
Italian, creamy	1 oz.	138
Low calorie	1 oz.	14
Oil & vinegar	1 oz.	124
Thousand Island	1 oz.	117
Shrimp dinner	7 pieces (3½ oz.)	220
Sirloin:		
Regular	3.3 oz. (edible portion)	220

Food and Description	Measure or Quantity	Calories
Super	6½ oz. (edible portion)	383
Tips	4 oz. (edible portion)	192
Steak sauce	1 oz.	23
Tartar sauce	1.5 oz.	285
T-Bone	4.3 oz. (edible portion)	240
Tomato (See also Salad Bar):		
Slices	2 slices (.9 oz.)	5
Whole, small	3.5 oz.	22
Topping, whipped	¼ oz.	19
Worcestershire sauce	1 tsp.	4
POPCORN:		
*Plain, popped fresh:		
(Jiffy Pop)	½ of 5-oz. pkg.	244
(Pillsbury) Microwave Popcorn:		
Regular	1 cup	70
Butter flavor	1 cup	65
Packaged:		
Buttered (Old London)	1 cup	57
Caramel-coated:		
(Bachman)	1-oz. serving	130
(Old London) without peanuts	1¾-oz. serving	195
Cheese flavored (Bachman)	1-oz. serving	180
Cracker Jack	¾-oz. serving	90
*POPOVER MIX (Flako)	1 popover	170
POPPY SEED (French's)	1 tsp.	13
POPSICLE, twin pop	3-fl. oz.	70
POP TARTS (See TOASTER CAKE OR PASTRY)		
PORK:		
Fresh:		
Chop:		
Broiled, lean & fat	3-oz. chop (weighed without bone)	332
Broiled, lean only	3-oz. chop (weighed without bone)	230
Loin:		
Roasted, lean & fat	3 oz.	308
Roasted, lean only	3 oz.	216
Spareribs, braised	3 oz.	246
Cured ham:		
Roasted, lean & fat	3 oz.	246
Roasted, lean only	3 oz.	159
PORK DINNER, frozen (Swanson)		
TV Brand	11¼-oz. dinner	270
PORK, PACKAGED (Eckrich)	1-oz. serving	45

Food and Description	Measure or Quantity	Calories
PORK RINDS, *Baken-Ets*	1-oz. serving	150
PORK STEAK, BREADED, FROZEN (Hormel)	3-oz. serving	223
PORK, SWEET & SOUR, frozen (La Choy)	½ of 15-oz. pkg.	229
PORT WINE:		
(Gallo)	3 fl. oz.	94
(Louis M. Martini)	3 fl. oz.	82
***POSTUM**, instant	6 fl. oz.	11
POTATO:		
Cooked:		
Au gratin	½ cup	127
Baked, peeled	2½″ dia. potato	92
Boiled, peeled	4.2-oz. potato	79
French-fried	10 pieces	156
Hash-browned, home recipe	½ cup	223
Mashed, milk & butter added	½ cup	92
Canned, solids & liq.:		
(Del Monte)	½ cup (4 oz.)	45
(Sunshine) whole	½ cup (4.1 oz.)	51
Frozen:		
(Birds Eye):		
Cottage fries	2.8-oz. serving	119
Crinkle cuts, regular	3-oz. serving	115
Farm style wedge	3-oz. serving	109
French fries, regular	3-oz. serving	113
Hash browns, shredded	¼ of 12-oz. pkg.	61
Steak fries	3-oz. serving	109
Tasti Puffs	¼ of 10-oz. pkg.	192
Tiny Taters	⅓ of 16-oz. pkg.	204
Whole, peeled	3.2 oz.	59
(Green Giant):		
Sliced, in butter sauce	½ cup	80
& sweet peas in bacon cream sauce	½ cup	110
(Stouffer's):		
Au gratin	⅓ of pkg.	135
Scalloped	⅓ of pkg.	125
POTATO & BACON, canned (Hormel) *Short Orders*, au gratin	7½-oz. can	240
POTATO & BEEF, canned, *Dinty Moore* (Hormel) *Short Orders*	1½-oz. can	250
POTATO CHIP:		
(Bachman) regular	1 oz.	160
(Featherweight) unsalted	1 oz.	160
(Frito-Lay's) natural	1 oz.	157
Lay's, sour cream & onion flavor	1 oz.	160

Food and Description	Measure or Quantity	Calories
Pringle's:		
Regular or *Cheez-Ums*	1 oz.	167
Light	1 oz.	148
POTATO & HAM, canned (Hormel)		
Short Orders, scalloped	7½-oz. can	250
***POTATO MIX:**		
Au gratin:		
(Betty Crocker)	½ cup	150
(French's) *Big Tate*, tangy	½ cup	150
(Libby's) *Potato Classics*	¾ cup	130
Creamed (Betty Crocker)	½ cup	160
Hash browns (Betty Crocker) with onion	½ cup	150
Hickory smoke cheese (Betty Crocker)	½ cup	150
Julienne (Betty Crocker) with mild cheese sauce	½ cup	130
Mashed:		
(American Beauty)	½ cup	120
(Betty Crocker) *Buds*	½ cup	130
(French's) *Big Tate*	½ cup	140
(Pillsbury) *Hungry Jack*, flakes	½ cup	140
Scalloped:		
(Betty Crocker)	½ cup	140
(French's) *Big Tate*	½ cup	160
(Libby's) *Potato Classics*	¾ cup	130
Sour cream & chive (Betty Crocker)	½ cup	150
***POTATO PANCAKE MIX**		
(French's) *Big Tate*	3″ pancake	43
POTATO SALAD:		
Home recipe	½ cup	181
Canned (Nalley's) German style	4-oz. serving	143
POTATO STICKS (Durkee) *O & C*	1½-oz. can	231
POTATO, STUFFED, BAKED, frozen (Green Giant):		
With cheese flavored topping	½ of 10-oz. pkg.	200
With sour cream & chives	½ of 10-oz. pkg.	230
POTATO TOPPERS (Libby's)	1 T.	30
POUND CAKE (See CAKE, Pound)		
PRESERVE OR JAM (See individual flavors):		
PRETZEL:		
(Bachman) regular or butter	1 oz.	110
(Estee) unsalted	1 piece	5
(Featherweight) unsalted	1 piece	7
(Nabisco) *Mister Salty*, Dutch	1 piece	55
PRODUCT 19, cereal (Kellogg's)	1 cup	110
PROSCIUTTO (Hormel) boneless	1 oz.	90

Food and Description	Measure or Quantity	Calories
PRUNE:		
Canned:		
(Featherweight) stewed,		
water pack	½ cup	130
(Sunsweet) stewed	½ cup	120
Dried:		
(Del Monte) Moist Pak	2 oz.	120
(Sunsweet) whole	2 oz.	130
PRUNE JUICE:		
(Del Monte)	6 fl. oz.	120
(Mott's) regular	6 fl. oz.	140
(Sunsweet) regular	6 fl. oz.	140
PRUNE NECTAR, canned (Mott's)	6 fl. oz.	100
PUDDING OR PIE FILLING:		
Canned, regular pack:		
Banana:		
(Del Monte) *Pudding Cup*	5-oz. container	181
(Hunt's) *Snack Pack*	5-oz. container	180
Butterscotch:		
(Del Monte) *Pudding Cup*	5-oz. container	184
(Hunt's) *Snack Pack*	5-oz. container	170
Chocolate:		
(Del Monte) *Pudding Cup*	5-oz. container	201
(Hunt's) *Snack Pack*	5-oz. container	180
Rice (Comstock; Menner's)	½ of 7½-oz. can	120
Tapioca:		
(Del Monte) *Pudding Cup*	5-oz. container	172
(Hunt's) *Snack Pack*	5-oz. container	140
Vanilla (Del Monte)	5-oz. container	188
Canned, dietetic pack (Sego)		
all flavors	4-oz. serving	125
Chilled, *Swiss Miss:*		
Butterscotch, chocolate malt		
or vanilla	4-oz. container	150
Chocolate or double rich	4-oz. container	160
Tapioca	4-oz. container	130
Frozen (Rich's):		
Banana	3-oz. container	142
Butterscotch or vanilla	4½-oz. container	199
Chocolate	4½-oz. container	214
*Mix, sweetened, regular & instant:		
Banana:		
(Jello-O) cream, regular	½ cup	161
(Royal) regular	½ cup	160
Butter pecan (Jello-O) instant	½ cup	175
Butterscotch:		
(Jell-O) instant	½ cup	175

Food and Description	Measure or Quantity	Calories
(My-T-Fine) regular	½ cup	143
(Royal)	½ cup	160
Chocolate:		
(Jell-O) regular	½ cup	174
(My-T-Fine) regular	½ cup	169
Coconut:		
(Jell-O) cream, regular	½ cup	176
(Royal) instant	½ cup	170
Custard (Royal) regular	½ cup	150
Flan (Royal) regular	½ cup	150
Lemon:		
(Jell-O) instant	½ cup	170
(My-T-Fine) regular	½ cup	164
Lime (Royal) Key Lime, regular	½ cup	160
Pineapple (Jell-O) cream, instant	½ cup	176
Pistachio (Jell-O) instant	½ cup	174
Raspberry (Salada)		
Danish Dessert	½ cup	176
Rice, Jell-O Americana	½ cup	176
Strawberry (Salada)		
Danish Dessert	½ cup	130
Tapioca:		
Jell-O Americana, chocolate	½ cup	173
(My-T-Fine) vanilla	½ cup	130
Vanilla:		
(Jell-O) French, regular	½ cup	172
(Royal)	½ cup	180
*Mix, dietetic:		
Butterscotch:		
(Dia-Mel)	½ cup	50
(D-Zerta)	½ cup	68
(Estee)	½ cup	70
(Featherweight) artificially sweetened	½ cup	60
Chocolate:		
(Dia-Mel)	½ cup	50
(D-Zerta)	½ cup	68
(Estee)	½ cup	70
Lemon:		
(Dia-Mel)	½ cup	53
(Estee)	½ cup	106
Vanilla:		
(Dia-Mel)	½ cup	50
(D-Zerta)	½ cup	71
(Estee)	½ cup	70
(Featherweight) artificially sweetened	½ cup	60

Food and Description	Measure or Quantity	Calories
PUFFED RICE:		
(Malt-O-Meal)	1 cup	50
(Quaker)	1 cup	55
PUFFED WHEAT:		
(Malt-O-Meal)	1 cup	50
(Quaker)	1 cup	54
PUMPKIN, canned (Libby's) solid pack	½ cup	80
PUMPKIN SEED, in hull	1 oz.	116

Q

Food and Description	Measure or Quantity	Calories
QUAIL, raw, meat & skin	4 oz.	195
QUIK, (Nestlé) chocolate or strawberry	1 tsp.	45
QUISP, cereal	1⅙ cup	121

R

Food and Description	Measure or Quantity	Calories
RADISH	2 small radishes	4
RAISIN, dried:		
(Del Monte) golden	3 oz.	260
(Sun-Maid)	1 oz.	290
RAISINS, RICE & RYE, cereal		
(Kellogg's)	¾ cup	140
RALSTON, cereal	¼ cup	90
RASPBERRY:		
Fresh:		
Black, trimmed	½ cup	49
Red, trimmed	½ cup	41
Frozen (Birds Eye) quick thaw	5-oz. serving	155
RASPBERRY PRESERVE OR JAM:		
Sweetened (Smucker's)	1 T.	53
Dietetic:		
(Dia-Mel, Louis Sherry)	1 T.	6
(Featherweight) red	1 T.	16
(S&W) *Nutradiet*, red	1 T.	12
RATATOUILLE, frozen (Stouffer's)	5-oz. serving	60
RAVIOLI:		
Canned, regular pack (Franco-American):		
Beef, *RavioliOs*	7½-oz. serving	120
Cheese, in tomato sauce, *RavioliOs*	8-oz. serving	214
Canned, dietetic (Dia-Mel) beef	8-oz. can	230
RELISH:		
Hamburger (Nally's)	1 T.	17
Hot dog (Nalley's)	1 T.	24
Sweet (Smucker's)	1 T.	23
RENNET MIX (Junket):		
*Powder, any flavor:		
Made with skim milk	½ cup	90
Made with whole milk	½ cup	120
Tablet	1 tablet	1
RHINE WINE:		
(Great Western)	3 fl. oz.	73
(Taylor)	3 fl. oz.	75
RHUBARB, cooked, sweetened	½ cup	169

Food and Description	Measure or Quantity	Calories
***RICE:**		
Brown (Uncle Ben's) parboiled, with added butter	⅔ cup	152
White:		
(Minute Rice) instant, no added butter	⅔ cup	120
(Success) long grain	½ cooking bag	110
White & wild (Carolina)	½ cup	90
RICE, FRIED (See also RICE MIX):		
*Canned (La Choy)	⅓ of 11-oz. can	190
Frozen:		
(Birds Eye)	3.7-oz. serving	104
(Green Giant) *Boil 'N Bag*	10-oz. entree	300
(La Choy) & pork	8-oz. serving	280
RICE, FRIED, SEASONING MIX (Kikkoman)	1-oz. pkg.	91
RICE KRINKLES, cereal(Post)	⅞ cup	109
RICE KRISPIES, cereal (Kellogg's)	1 cup	110
RICE MIX:		
Beef:		
*(Carolina) *Bake-It-Easy*	¼ of pkg.	110
(Minute Rice)	½ cup	149
Rice-A-Roni	⅙ of 8-oz. pkg.	129
Chicken:		
*(Carolina) *Bake-It-Easy*	¼ of pkg.	110
Rice-A-Roni	⅕ of 8-oz. pkg.	160
*Fried (Minute Rice)	½ cup	156
*Long grain & wild (Minute Rice)	½ cup	148
*Oriental (Carolina) *Bake-It-Easy*	½ of pkg.	120
Spanish:		
*(Carolina) *Bake-It-Easy*	¼ of pkg.	110
*(Minute Rice)	½ cup	150
Rice-A-Roni	⅙ of 7½-oz. pkg.	124
RICE, SPANISH, canned:		
Regular pack (Comstock; Menner's)	½ of 7½-oz. can	140
Dietetic (Featherweight) low sodium	7½-oz. serving	140
Frozen (Birds Eye)	3.7-oz. serving	122
RICE & VEGETABLE, frozen:		
(Birds Eye):		
French style	3.7-oz. serving	117
Peas with mushrooms	2⅓ oz.	109
(Green Giant) *Rice Originals*		
& broccoli in cheese sauce	½ cup	140
& herb butter sauce	½ cup	150
Pilaf	½ cup	120
RICE WINE:		
Chinese, 20.7% alcohol	1 fl. oz.	38
Japanese, 10.6% alcohol	1 fl. oz.	72

Food and Description	Measure or Quantity	Calories
ROCK & RYE (Mr. Boston)	1 fl. oz.	74
ROE, baked or broiled, cod & shad	4 oz.	143
ROLL OR BUN:		
Commercial type, non-frozen:		
Biscuit (Wonder)	1¼-oz. piece	80
Brown & serve (Wonder)		
Gem Style	1-oz. piece	80
Club (Pepperidge Farm)	1.3-oz. piece	100
Crescent (Pepperidge Farm)		
butter	1-oz. piece	110
Croissant (Pepperidge Farm):		
Butter, cinnamon or		
honey-sesame	2-oz. piece	200
Chocolate	2.4-oz. piece	260
Walnut	2-oz. piece	210
Dinner:		
Home Pride	1-oz. piece	85
(Pepperidge Farm)	.7-oz. piece	60
Finger (Pepperidge Farm) sesame		
or poppy seed	.6-oz. piece	60
Frankfurter:		
(Arnold) Hot Dog	1.3-oz. piece	100
(Pepperidge Farm)	1¾-oz. piece	110
(Wonder)	1-oz. piece	80
French:		
(Arnold) *Francisco*, sourdough	1.1-oz. piece	90
(Pepperidge Farm):		
Small	1.3-oz. piece	110
Large	3-oz. piece	240
Golden Twist (Pepperidge Farm)	1-oz. piece	120
Hamburger:		
(Arnold)	1.4-oz. piece	110
(Pepperidge Farm)	1.5-oz. piece	130
Roman Meal	1.8-oz. piece	193
Hoagie (Wonder)	5-oz. piece	400
Old fashioned (Pepperidge Farm)	.6-oz. piece	60
Parkerhouse (Pepperidge Farm)	.6-oz. piece	60
Party (Pepperidge Farm)	.4-oz. piece	45
Sandwich (Arnold) soft	1.3-oz. piece	110
Soft (Pepperidge Farm)	1¼-oz. piece	110
Frozen:		
Apple crunch (Sara Lee)	1-oz. piece	102
Caramel pecan (Sara Lee)	1.3-oz. piece	161
Cinnamon (Sara Lee)	.9-oz. piece	100
Croissant (Sara Lee)	.9-oz. piece	109
Crumb (Sara Lee) French	1¾-oz. piece	188

Food and Description	Measure or Quantity	Calories
Danish (Sara Lee):		
Apple	1.3-oz. piece	120
Cheese	1.3-oz. piece	130
Cinnamon raisin	1.3-oz. piece	147
Pecan	1.3-oz. piece	148
Honey (Morton) mini	1.3-oz. piece	133
*ROLL OR BUN DOUGH:		
Frozen (Rich's):		
Cinnamon	2¼-oz. piece	173
Frankfurter	1 piece	136
Hamburger, regular	1 piece	134
Parkerhouse	1 piece	82
Refrigerated (Pillsbury):		
Apple danish, *Pipin' Hot*	1 piece	250
Caramel danish, with nuts	1 piece	155
Cinnamon raisin danish	1 piece	145
Crescent	1 piece	100
White, bakery style	1 piece	100
*ROLL MIX, HOT (Pillsbury)	1 piece	100
ROMAN MEAL CEREAL	⅓ cup	103
ROSEMARY LEAVES (French's)	1 tsp.	103
ROSÉ WINE:		
(Great Western)	3 fl. oz.	80
(Paul Masson):		
Regular, 11.8% alcohol	3 fl. oz.	76
Light. 7.1% alcohol	3 fl. oz.	49
RUTABAGA:		
Canned (Sunshine) solids & liq.	½ cup	32
Frozen (Sunshine)	4 oz.	50

S

Food and Description	Measure or Quantity	Calories
SAFFLOWER SEED, in hull	1 oz.	89
SAGE (French's)	1 tsp.	4
SAKE WINE	1 fl. oz.	39
SALAD CRUNCHIES (Libby's)	1 T.	35
SALAD DRESSING:		
Regular:		
Bacon (Seven Seas) creamy	1 T.	60
Bleu or blue cheese:		
(Bernstein) Danish	1 T.	60
(Wish-Bone) chunk	1 T.	70
Caesar:		
(Pfeiffer)	1 T.	70
(Seven Seas) *Viva*	1 T.	60
Capri (Seven Seas)	1 T.	70
Cheddar & bacon (Wish-Bone)	1 T.	70
Cucumber (Wish-Bone)	1 T.	80
French:		
(Bernstein's) creamy	1 T.	56
(Seven Seas) creamy	1 T.	60
(Wish-Bone) garlic or herbal	1 T.	60
Garlic (Wish-Bone) creamy	1 T.	80
Green Goddess:		
(Seven Seas)	1 T.	60
(Wish-Bone)	1 T.	70
Herb & spice (Seven Seas)	1 T.	60
Italian:		
(Bernstein's)	1 T.	50
(Pfeiffer) chef	1 T.	60
(Seven Seas) *VIVA!*	1 T.	70
(Wish-Bone) regular, creamy or robusto	1 T.	80
Red wine vinegar & oil (Seven Seas)	1 T.	60
Roquefort:		
(Bernstein's)	1 T.	65
(Marie's)	1 T.	105
Russian:		
(Pfeiffer)	1 T.	65
(Wish-Bone)	1 T.	50
Spin Blend (Hellmann's)	1 T.	57

111

Food and Description	Measure or Quantity	Calories
Thousand Island:		
(Pfeiffer)	1 T.	65
(Wish-Bone)	1 T.	70
Vinaigrette (Bernstein's) French	1 T.	49
Dietetic or low calorie:		
Bleu or blue cheese:		
(Dia-Mel)	1 T.	2
(Featherweight) imitation	1 T.	4
(Tillie Lewis) *Tasti-Diet*	1 T.	12
(Walden Farms) chunky	1 T.	27
(Wish-Bone) chunky	1 T.	40
Caesar:		
(Estee) garlic	1 T.	4
(Featherweight) creamy	1 T.	14
Cucumber (Dia-Mel) creamy	1 T.	2
Cucumber (Wish-Bone) creamy	1 T.	40
French:		
(Dia-Mel)	1 T.	1
(Featherweight) low calorie	1 T.	6
(Walden Farms)	1 T.	33
(Wish-Bone)	1 T.	30
Herb & spice (Featherweight)	1 T.	6
Garlic (Dia-Mel)	1 T.	1
Italian:		
(Dia-Mel)	1 T.	1
(Estee) spicy	1 T.	4
(Walden Farm) regular	1 T.	9
(Weight Watchers)	1 T.	50
(Wish-Bone)	1 T.	30
Onion & chive (Wish-Bone)	1 T.	40
Onion & cucumber (Estee)	1 T.	6
Red wine/vinegar (Featherweight)	1 T.	6
Russian:		
(Featherweight) creamy	1 T.	6
(Weight Watchers)	1 T.	50
(Wish-Bone)	1 T.	25
Tahiti (Dia-Mel)	1 T.	2
Thousand Island:		
(Dia-Mel)	1 T.	2
(Walden Farms)	1 T.	24
(Weight Watchers)	1 T.	50
(Wish-Bone)	1 T.	25
2-Calorie Low Sodium		
(Featherweight)	1 T.	2
Whipped (Tillie Lewis) *Tasti Diet*	1 T.	18
Yogurt-buttermilk (Dia-Mel)	1 T.	2

Food and Description	Measure or Quantity	Calories
SALAD DRESSING MIX:		
*Regular (Good Seasons):		
Blue cheese	1 T.	84
Buttermilk, farm style	1 T.	58
Farm style	1 T.	53
French, old fashioned	1 T.	83
Garlic, cheese	1 T.	85
Garlic & herb	1 T.	84
Italian, regular, cheese or zesty	1 T.	84
Dietetic:		
*Blue cheese (Weight Watchers)	1 T.	10
*French (Weight Watchers)	1 T.	4
Garlic (Dia-Mel)	½-oz. pkg.	21
*Italian:		
(Good Seasons) regular	1 T.	8
(Weight Watchers):		
Regular	1 T.	2
Creamy	1 T.	4
*Russian (Weight Watchers)	1 T.	4
*Thousand Island		
(Weight Watchers)	1 T.	12
SALAD SUPREME (McCormick)	1 tsp.	11
SALAMI:		
(Eckrich) for beer or cooked	1 oz.	70
(Hormel):		
Beef	1 slice	40
Genoa, DiLusso	1-oz. serving	100
Hard, sliced	1-slice	40
(Oscar Mayer):		
For beer, beef	.8-oz. slice	76
Cotto	.8-oz. slice	52
SALISBURY STEAK, frozen:		
(Banquet):		
Buffet Supper	2-lb. pkg.	1410
Man Pleaser	19-oz. dinner	1024
(Green Giant) with gravy, oven bake	7-oz. serving	280
(Morton) *Country Table*	15-oz. dinner	500
(Stouffer's) *Lean Cuisine*	9½-oz. pkg.	270
(Swanson):		
Regular, with gravy	10-oz. entree	410
Hungry Man	17-oz. dinner	780
TV Brand	11½-oz. dinner	430
SALMON:		
Baked or broiled	6¾" × 2½" × 1" piece	264
Canned, regular pack, solids & liq.:		
Keta (Bumble Bee)	½ cup	153

113

Food and Description	Measure or Quantity	Calories
Pink or Humpback:		
(Bumble Bee)	½ cup	155
(Del Monte)	7¾-oz. can	290
Sockeye or Red or Blueback:		
(Bumble Bee)	½ cup	188
(Libby's)	7¾-oz. can	380
Canned, dietetic (S&W) *Nutradiet*, low sodium	½ cup	188
SALMON, SMOKED (Vita):		
Lox, drained	4-oz. jar	136
Nova, drained	4-oz. can	221
SALT:		
(Morton):		
Regular	1 tsp.	0
Lite	1 tsp.	0
Substitute:		
(Adolph's) plain	1 tsp.	1
(Morton) plain	1 tsp.	Tr.
Salt-It (Dia-Mel)	1 tsp.	0
SALT 'N SPICE SEASONING (McCormick)	1 tsp.	3
SANDWICH SPREAD:		
(Hellmann's)	1 T.	65
(Oscar Mayer)	1-oz. serving	68
SANGRIA (Taylor)	3 fl. oz.	99
SARDINE, canned:		
Atlantic (Del Monte) with tomato sauce	7½-oz. can	319
Imported (Underwood) in mustard or tomato sauce	3¾-oz. can	230
Norwegian, *King Oscar Brand:*		
In mustard or tomato sauce	3¾-oz. can	240
In oil, drained	3-oz. can	260
SAUCE:		
Regular:		
A-1	1 T.	12
Barbecue:		
Chris & Pitt's	1 T.	15
(Gold's)	1 T.	25
Open Pit (General Foods) original, hot n' spicy or smoke flavor	1 T.	24
Burrito (DelMonte)	¼ cup	20
Chili (See CHILI SAUCE)		
Cocktail:		
(Gold's)	1 T.	31
(Pfeiffer)	1-oz. serving	100
Escoffier Sauce Diable	1 T.	20

Food and Description	Measure or Quantity	Calories
Escoffier Sauce Robert	1 T.	20
Famous Sauce	1 T.	69
Hot, *Frank's*	1 tsp.	1
Italian (See also SPAGHETTI SAUCE or TOMATO SAUCE):		
(Contadina)	4-oz. serving	71
(Ragu) red cooking	3½-oz. serving	45
Salsa Mexicana (Contadina)	4 fl. oz.	38
Salsa Picante (Del Monte) regular	¼ cup	20
Salsa Roja (Del Monte)	¼ cup	20
Seafood cocktail (Del Monte)	1 T.	21
Soy:		
(Gold's)	1 T.	10
(Kikkoman) light	1 T.	9
(La Choy)	1 T.	8
Spare rib (Gold's)	1 T.	51
Steak (Dawn Fresh) with mushrooms	1-oz. serving	9
Steak Supreme	1 T.	20
Sweet & sour:		
(Contadina)	4 fl. oz.	150
(La Choy)	1-oz. serving	51
Swiss steak (Carnation)	2-oz. serving	20
Tabasco	¼ tsp.	Tr.
Taco:		
Old El Paso	1-oz. serving	10
(Ortega)	1 T.	22
Tartar:		
(Hellmann's)	1 T.	73
(Nalley's)	1 T.	89
Teriyaki (Kikkoman)	1 T.	16
V-8	1-oz. serving	25
White, medium	¼ cup	103
Worcestershire:		
(French's) regular or smoky	1 T.	10
(Gold's)	1 T.	42
Dietetic (Estee):		
Barbecue	1 T.	16
Cocktail	1 T.	10
SAUCE MIX:		
Regular:		
A la King (Durkee)	1-oz. pkg.	133
*Cheese:		
(Durkee)	½ cup	168
(French's)	½ cup	160
Hollandaise:		
(Durkee)	1 oz. pkg.	173
*(French's)	1 T.	15

Food and Description	Measure or Quantity	Calories
*Sour cream (French's)	2½ T.	60
Sweet & sour (Kikkoman)	2⅛-oz. pkg.	228
Teriyaki (Kikkoman)	1.5-oz. pkg.	125
*White (Durkee)	1 cup	238
*Dietetic (Weight Watchers) lemon butter	1 T.	8
SAUERKRAUT, canned:		
(Claussen) drained	½ cup	16
(Del Monte) solids & liq.	1 cup	55
(Silver Floss) solids & liq.:		
Regular	½ cup	30
Krispy Kraut	½ cup	25
SAUSAGE:		
*Brown & serve (Hormel)	1 sausage	70
Patty (Hormel)	1 patty	150
Polish-style (Eckrich)	1-oz. serving	95
Pork:		
(Eckrich)	1-oz. link	100
*(Hormel) *Litte Sizzlers*	1 link	51
(Jimmy Dean)	2-oz. serving	227
*(Oscar Mayer) *Little Friers*	.6-oz. link	64
Roll (Eckrich) minced	1-oz. slice	80
Smoked:		
(Eckrich) beef, *Smok-Y-Links*	.8-oz. link	70
(Hormel) smokies	1 sausage	80
(Oscar Mayer) beef	1½-oz. link	132
*Turkey (Louis Rich) links or tube	1-oz. serving	45
Vienna:		
(Hormel) regular	1 sausage	50
(Libby's) in barbecue sauce	2½-oz. serving	180
SAUTERNE:		
(Great Western)	3 fl. oz.	79
(Taylor)	3 fl. oz.	81
SCALLOP:		
Steamed	4-oz. serving	127
Frozen:		
(Mrs. Paul's) breaded & fried	3½-oz. serving	210
(Stouffer's) *Lean Cuisine*	*11-oz. pkg.*	230
SCHNAPPS, APPLE (Mr. Boston)	1 fl. oz.	76
SCHNAPPS, PEPPERMINT (Mr. Boston)	1 fl. oz.	115
SCREWDRIVER COCKTAIL (Mr. Boston) 12½% alcohol	3 fl. oz.	111
SEAFOOD PLATTER, frozen (Mrs. Paul's) breaded & fried	9-oz. serving	510
SEGO DIET FOOD, canned, any flavor	10-fl.-oz. can	225
SELTZER (Canada Dry)	Any quantity	0

116

Food and Description	Measure or Quantity	Calories
SERUTAN	1 tsp.	6
SESAME SEEDS (French's)	1 tsp.	9
SHAD, CREOLE	4-oz. serving	172
SHAKE 'N BAKE:		
Chicken, original	1 pkg.	282
Crispy country mild	1 pkg.	309
Fish	2-oz. pkg.	232
Italian	1 pkg.	289
Pork, barbecue	1 pkg.	306
SHELLS, PASTA, STUFFED		
(Stouffer's) cheese stuffed	9-oz. serving	320
SHERBET:		
(Baskin-Robbins):		
Daiquiri Ice	1 scoop	84
Orange	1 scoop	99
(Howard Johnson's)	½ cup	132
(Meadow Gold) orange	¼ pint	120
SHERRY:		
Cocktail (Gold Seal)	3 fl. oz.	122
Cream (Great Western) Solera	3 fl. oz.	141
Dry (Williams & Humbert)	3 fl. oz.	120
Dry Sack (Williams &Humbert)	3 fl. oz.	120
SHREDDED WHEAT:		
(Nabisco):		
Regular size	¾-oz. biscuit	90
Spoon Size	⅔ cup	110
(Quaker)	1 biscuit	52
SHRIMP:		
Canned (Bumble Bee) solids & liq.	4½oz. can	90
Frozen (Mrs. Paul's) fried	3-oz. serving	190
SHRIMP DINNER, frozen:		
(Stouffer's) Newburg	6½-oz. serving	300
(Van de Kamp's)	10-oz. dinner	370
SLENDER (Carnation):		
Bar	1 bar	135
Dry	1 packet	110
Liquid	10-fl.-oz. can	220
SLOPPY HOT DOG SEASONING MIX (French's)	1½-oz. pkg.	160
SLOPPY JOE:		
Canned:		
(Hormel) *Short Orders*	7½-oz. can	340
(Libby's):		
Beef	⅓ cup	110
Pork	⅓ cup	120
Frozen (Banquet) *Cookin' Bag*	5-oz. pkg.	199
SLOPPY JOE SEASONING MIX:		
*(Durkee) pizza flavor	1¼ cups	746

Food and Description	Measure or Quantity	Calories
(French's)	1.5-oz. pkg.	128
(McCormick)	1.3-oz. pkg.	103
SMURF BERRY CRUNCH, cereal		
(Post)	1 cup	116
SNACK BAR (Pepperidge Farm):		
Apple nut, apricot-raspberry		
or blueberry	1.7-oz. piece	170
Brownie nut or date nut	1½-oz. piece	190
Chocolate chip or coconut macaroon	1½-oz. piece	210
SNO BALL (Hostess)	1 piece	149
SOAVE WINE (Antinori)	3 fl. oz.	84
SOFT DRINK		
Sweetened:		
Birch beer (Canada Dry)	6 fl. oz.	82
Bitter lemon:		
(Canada Dry)	6 fl. oz.	75
(Schweppes)	6 fl. oz.	84
Bubble Up	6 fl. oz.	73
Cactus Cooler (Canada Dry)	6 fl. oz.	90
Cherry:		
(Canada Dry) wild	6 fl. oz.	98
(Shasta) black	6 fl. oz.	79
Chocolate (Yoo-Hoo)	6 fl. oz.	93
Club	Any qantity	0
Cola:		
Coca-Cola:		
Regular	6 fl. oz.	72
Caffeine-free	6 fl. oz.	76
Jamaica (Canada Dry)	6 fl. oz.	79
Pepsi-Cola, regular or		
Pepsi Free	6 fl. oz.	79
(Shasta)	6 fl. oz.	72
Collins mix (Canada Dry)	6 fl. oz.	60
Cream:		
(Canada Dry) vanilla	6 fl. oz.	97
(Schweppes) red	6 fl. oz.	86
(Shasta)	6 fl. oz.	75
Dr. Pepper	6 fl. oz.	75
Fruit punch:		
(Nehi)	6 fl. oz.	91
(Shasta)	6 fl. oz.	84
Ginger ale:		
(Canada Dry) regular	6 fl. oz.	68
(Fanta)	6 fl. oz.	63
(Shasta)	6 fl. oz.	59
Ginger beer (Schweppes)	6 fl. oz.	72
Grape:		
(Canada Dry) concord	6 fl. oz.	97

Food and Description	Measure or Quantity	Calories
(Fanta; Nehi)	6 fl. oz.	86
(Hi-C)	6 fl. oz.	78
(Schweppes)	6 fl. oz.	97
(Welch's) sparkling	6 fl. oz.	90
Half & half (Canada Dry)	6 fl. oz.	82
Hi-Spot (Canada Dry)	6 fl. oz.	75
Lemon (Hi-C)	6 fl. oz.	75
Mello Yello	6 fl. oz.	86
Mountain Dew	6 fl. oz.	89
Mr. PiBB	6 fl. oz.	71
Orange:		
(Canada Dry) *Sunrise*	6 fl. oz.	97
(Hi-C)	6 fl. oz.	77
(Sunkist)	6 fl. oz.	96
Peach (Nehi)	6 fl. oz.	92
Pineapple (Canada Dry)	6 fl. oz.	82
Quinine or tonic water		
(Canada Dry; Schweppes)	6 fl. oz.	66
Root beer:		
Barrelhead (Canada Dry)	6 fl. oz.	82
(Dad's)	6 fl. oz.	83
Rooti (Canada Dry)	6 fl. oz.	79
(Shasta) draft	6 fl. oz.	75
Seven-Up	6 fl. oz.	60
Sprite	6 fl. oz.	71
Strawberry (Shasta)	6 fl. oz.	72
Tahitian Treat (Canada Dry)	6 fl. oz.	97
Upper Ten (Royal Crown)	6 fl. oz.	76
Wink (Canada Dry)	6 fl. oz.	90
Dietetic:		
Bubble Up	6 fl. oz.	1
Cherry (Shasta) black	6 fl. oz.	<1
Chocolate (No-Cal)	6 fl. oz.	1
Coffee (No-Cal)	6 fl. oz.	1
Cola:		
(Canada Dry; No-Cal)	6 fl. oz.	0
Coca-Cola, regular or caffeine free	6 fl. oz.	<1
Diet Rite	6 fl. oz.	<1
Pepsi, diet, light or caffeine free	6 fl. oz.	<1
Cream (Shasta)	6 fl. oz.	<1
Dr. Pepper	6 fl. oz.	<2
Fresca	6 fl. oz.	2
Ginger Ale:		
(Canada Dry)	6 fl. oz.	1
(No-Cal)	6 fl. oz.	0
Grape (Shasta)	6 fl. oz.	<1

Food and Description	Measure or Quantity	Calories
Grapefruit (Shasta)	6 fl. oz.	<1
Mr. PiBB	6 fl. oz.	<1
Orange:		
(Canada Dry; No-Cal)	6 fl. oz.	1
(Shasta)	6 fl. oz.	<1
Quinine or tonic (No-Cal)	6 fl. oz.	3
RC 100 (Royal Crown)		
caffeine free	6 fl. oz.	<1
Root beer:		
Barrelhead (Canada Dry)	6 fl. oz.	1
(Dad's; Ramblin'; Shasta)	6 fl. oz.	<1
Seven-Up	6 fl. oz.	2
Sprite	6 fl. oz.	1
Tab, regular or caffeine free	6 fl. oz.	<1
SOLE, frozen:		
(Mrs. Paul's) fillets,		
breaded & fried	6-oz. serving	280
(Van De Kamp's) batter dipped,		
french fried	1 piece	140
(Weight Watchers) in lemon sauce	9⅛-oz. meal	200
SOUFFLE, frozen (Stouffer's):		
Cheese	6-oz. serving	355
Corn	4-oz. serving	155
SOUP:		
Canned, regular pack:		
*Asparagus (Campbell),		
condensed, cream of	8-oz. serving	90
Bean:		
(Campbell):		
Chunky, with ham,		
old fashioned	11-oz. can	290
*Condensed, with bacon	8-oz. serving	150
(Grandma Brown's)	8-oz. serving	182
Bean, black:		
*(Campbell) condensed	8-oz. serving	110
(Crosse & Blackwell)	6½-oz. serving	80
Beef:		
(Campbell):		
Chunky:		
Regular	10¾-oz. can	190
With noodles	10¾-oz. can	300
*Condensed:		
Regular	8-oz. serving	80
Broth, & noodles	8-oz. serving	60
Consomme	8-oz. serving	25
Noodle	8-oz. serving	70
Teriyaki	8-oz. serving	70

Food and Description	Measure or Quantity	Calories
(College Inn) broth	1 cup	18
(Swanson)	7½-oz. can	20
Celery:		
*(Campbell) condensed, cream of	8-oz. serving	100
*(Rokeach):		
Prepared with milk	10-oz. serving	190
Prepared with water	10-oz. serving	90
*Cheddar cheese (Campbell)	8-oz. serving	130
Chicken:		
(Campbell):		
Chunky:		
Regular	10¾-oz. can	200
& rice	19-oz. can	280
vegetable	19-oz. can	340
*Condensed:		
Alphabet	8-oz. serving	80
Broth:		
Plain	8-oz. serving	35
& rice	8-oz. serving	50
Cream of	8-oz. serving	110
Mushroom, creamy	8-oz. serving	110
NoodleOs	8-oz. serving	70
& rice	8-oz. serving	·60
Vegetable	8-oz. serving	70
*Semi-condensed,		
Soup For One,		
vegetable, full flavored	11-oz. serving	120
(College Inn) broth	1 cup	35
(Swanson) broth	7¼-oz. can	35
Chili beef (Campbell) *Chunky*	11-oz. can	300
Chowder:		
Beef'n vegetable (Hormel) *Short Orders*	7½-oz. can	120
Chicken'n corn (Hormel) *Short Orders*	7½-oz. can	130
Clam:		
Manhattan style:		
(Campbell):		
Chunky	19-oz. can	300
*Condensed	8-oz. serving	70
(Crosse & Blackwell)	6½-oz. serving	50
New England style:		
*(Campbell):		
Condensed:		
Made with milk	8-oz. serving	150
Made with water	8-oz. serving	80

Food and Description	Measure or Quantity	Calories
Semi-condensed, *Soup for One:*		
Make with milk	11-oz. serving	200
Made with water	11-oz. serving	130
(Crosse & Blackwell)	6½-oz. serving	90
Ham'n potato (Hormel)	7½-oz. can	130
Consomme madrilene		
(Crosse & Blackwell)	6½-oz. serving	25
Crab (Crosse & Blackwell)	6½-oz. serving	50
Gazpacho (Crosse & Blackwell)	6½-oz. serving	30
Ham'n butter bean (Campbell) *Chunky*	10¾-oz. can	280
Lentil (Crosse & Blackwell) with ham	6½-oz. serving	80
*Meatball alphabet (Campbell) condensed	8-oz. serving	100
Minestrone:		
(Campbell):		
Chunky	19-oz. can	300
*Condensed	8-oz. serving	80
(Crosse & Blackwell)	6½-oz. serving	90
Mushroom:		
*(Campbell):		
Condensed:		
Cream of	8-oz. serving	100
Golden	8-oz. serving	80
Semi-condensed, *Soup For One,* cream of, savory	11-oz. serving	180
(Crosse & Blackwell) cream of, bisque	6½-oz. serving	90
*(Rokeach) cream of		
Prepared with milk	10-oz. serving	240
Prepared with water	10-oz. serving	150
*Mushroom barley (Campbell)	8-oz. serving	80
*Noodle (Campbell) & ground beef	8-oz. serving	90
*Onion (Campbell):		
Regular	8-oz. serving	70
Cream of:		
Made with water	8-oz. serving	100
Made with water & milk	8-oz. serving	160
*Oyster stew (Campbell):		
Made with milk	8-oz. serving	140
Made with water	8-oz. serving	70
*Pea, green (Campbell)	8-oz. serving	150

Food and Description	Measure or Quantity	Calories
Pea, split:		
(Campbell):		
Chunky, with ham	19-oz. can	400
*Condensed, with		
ham & bacon	8-oz. serving	170
(Grandma Brown's)	8-oz. serving	184
*Pepper pot (Campbell)	8-oz. serving	90
*Potato (Campbell) cream of:		
Made with water	8-oz. serving	70
Made with water & milk	8-oz. serving	130
Shav (Gold's)	8-oz. serving	11
Shrimp:		
*(Campbell) condensed, cream of:		
Made with milk	8-oz. serving	160
Made with water	8-oz. serving	90
(Crosse & Blackwell)	6½-oz. serving	90
Steak & potato (Campbell) *Chunky*	19-oz. can	340
Tomato:		
(Campbell):		
Condensed:		
Regular:		
Made with milk	8-oz. serving	160
Made with water	8-oz. serving	90
& rice, old fashioned	8-oz. serving	110
Semi-condensed,		
Soup For One, Royale	11-oz. serving	180
*(Rokeach):		
Made with milk	10-oz. serving	190
Made with water	10-oz. serving	90
Turkey (Campbell) *Chunky*	18¾-oz. can	360
Vegetable:		
(Campbell):		
Chunky:		
Regular	19-oz. can	260
Beef, old fashioned	19-oz. can	360
*Condensed:		
Regular	8-oz. serving	80
Beef or vegetarian	10-oz. serving	70
*Semi-condensed,		
Soup For One, old world	11-oz. serving	130
*(Rokeach) vegetarian	10-oz. serving	90
Vichyssoise (Crosse & Blackwell)	6½-oz. serving	70
*Won ton (Campbell)	8-oz. serving	40
Canned, dietetic pack:		
Beef (Campbell) *Chunky,* & mushroom, low sodium	10¾-oz. can	200

Food and Description	Measure or Quantity	Calories
Chicken:		
(Campbell) low sodium:		
Chunky, regular	7½-oz. can	150
Vegetable	10¾-oz. can	240
*(Dia-Mel) & noodle	8-oz. serving	50
Mushroom (Campbell) cream of, low sodium	7¼-oz. can	130
Pea, green (Cambell) low sodium	7½-oz. can	160
Pea, split (Campbell) low sodium	10¾-oz. can	220
Tomato:		
(Campbell) low sodium:		
Regular	7¼-oz. can	140
With tomato pieces	10½-oz. can	200
(Dia-Mel)	8-oz. serving	50
Vegetable (Campbell) low sodium, regular	7¼-oz. can	90
Frozen:		
*Barley & mushroom (Mother's Own)	8-oz. serving	50
Chowder, clam, New England style (Stouffer's)	8-oz. serving	200
Pea, split:		
*(Mother's Own)	8-oz. serving	130
(Stouffer's)	8¼-oz. serving	190
Spinach (Stouffer's) cream of	8-oz. serving	230
*Won ton (La Choy)	½ of 15-oz. pkg.	50
Mix, regular:		
Beef:		
*Caramel Kosher	6 fl. oz.	12
*(Lipton) *Cup-A-Soup*, regular & noodle	6 fl. oz.	45
*(Weight Watchers) broth	6 fl. oz.	10
*Chicken:		
Carmel Kosher	6 fl. oz.	12
(Lipton):		
Cup-A-Broth	6 fl. oz.	25
Cup-A-Soup, & rice	6 fl. oz.	45
Country style, hearty	6 fl. oz.	70
Lots-A-Noodles	7 fl. oz.	120
*Noodle (Lipton):		
With chicken broth	8 fl. oz.	70
With chicken meat	8 fl. oz.	50
*Mushroom:		
Carmel Kosher	6 fl. oz.	12
(Lipton):		
Regular, beef	8 fl. oz.	40
Cup-A-Soup, cream of	6 fl. oz.	80

Food and Description	Measure or Quantity	Calories
*Onion:		
Carmel Kosher	6 fl. oz.	12
(Lipton):		
Regular, beef	8 fl. oz.	35
Cup-A-Soup	6 fl. oz.	30
*Pea, green (Lipton) *Cup-A-Soup*	6 fl. oz.	120
*Tomato (Lipton) *Cup-A-Soup*	6 fl. oz.	80
*Vegetable:		
(Lipton):		
Regular, country	8 fl. oz.	80
Cup-A-Soup:		
Regular, spring	6 fl. oz.	40
Country style, harvest	6 fl. oz.	90
Lots-A-Noodles, garden	7 fl. oz.	130
(Southland) frozen	⅓ of 16-oz. pkg.	60
*Mix, dietetic (Estee)		
cream of chicken or mushroom	6½-oz. serving	50
SOUP GREENS (Durkee)	2⅓-oz. jar	216
SOUTHERN COMFORT:		
86 proof	1 fl. oz.	84
100 proof	1 fl. oz.	96
SOYBEAN CURD OR TOFU	2¾" × 1½" × 1"cake	86
SOYBEAN OR NUT:		
Dry roasted (*Soy Ahoy: Soy Town*)	1 oz.	139
Oil roasted (*Soy Ahoy; Soy Town*)		
plain, barbecue or garlic	1 oz.	152
SPAGHETTI:		
Cooked:		
8-10 minutes, "Al Dente"	1 cup	216
14-20 minutes, tender	1 cup	155
Canned:		
(Franco-American):		
With meatballs in tomato sauce,		
SpaghettiOs	7⅜-oz. can	220
In meat sauce	7½-oz. can	220
With sliced franks in		
tomato sauce, *SpaghettiOs*	7⅜-oz. can	220
In tomato sauce with cheese	7⅜-oz. can	180
(Hormel) *Short Orders,* &		
meatballs in tomato sauce	7½-oz. can	210
(Libby's) & meatballs in		
tomato sauce	7½-oz. serving	189
Dietetic (Dia-Mel) & meatballs	8-oz. serving	220
Frozen:		
(Banquet) & meat sauce	8-oz. pkg.	270
(Morton) & meatball	11-oz. dinner	360
(Stouffer's) *Lean Cuisine*	11½-oz. pkg.	280
(Swanson) *TV Brand*	12½-oz. dinner	370

Food and Description	Measure or Quantity	Calories
SPAGHETTI SAUCE, CANNED:		
Regular pack:		
Garden Style (Ragu)	4-oz. serving	80
Marinara:		
(Prince)	4-oz. serving	80
(Ragu)	5-oz. serving	120
Meat or meat flavored:		
(Prego)	4-oz. serving	160
(Prince)	½ cup	101
(Ragu) regular	4-oz. serving	80
Meatless or plain:		
(Prego)	4-oz. serving	160
(Prince)	½ cup	90
(Ragu) regular	4-oz. serving	80
Mushroom:		
(Hain)	4-oz. serving	80
(Prego)	4-oz. serving	140
(Prince)	4-oz. serving	77
(Ragu) Extra Thick & Zesty	4-oz. serving	110
Dietetic pack (Featherweight)	⅔ cup	30
*SPAGHETTI SAUCE MIX:		
(Durkee) regular	½ cup	45
(French's) with mushrooms	⅝ cup	100
(Spatini)	½ cup	84
SPAM, luncheon meat (Hormel):		
Regular, smoke flavored or with cheese chunks	1-oz. serving	85
Deviled	1 T.	35
SPECIAL K, cereal (Kellogg's)	1 cup	110
SPINACH:		
Fresh, whole leaves	½ cup	4
Boiled	½ cup	18
Canned, regular pack (Sunshine) solids & liq.	½ cup	24
Canned, dietetic pack (Del Monte) No Salt Added	½ cup	25
Frozen:		
(Birds Eye):		
Chopped or leaf	⅓ of pkg.	28
Creamed	⅓ of pkg.	60
(Green Giant):		
Creamed	½ cup	70
Harvest Fresh	4-oz. serving	30
(McKenzie) chopped or cut	⅓ of pkg.	20
(Stouffer's) souffle	4-oz. serving	135
SQUASH, SUMMER:		
Yellow, boiled slices	½ cup	13
Zucchini, boiled slices	½ cup	9

Food and Description	Measure or Quantity	Calories
Canned (Del Monte) zucchini, in tomato sauce	½ cup	30
Frozen:		
(Birds Eye) zucchini	⅓ of pkg.	19
(McKenzie) crookneck	⅓ of pkg.	18
(Mrs. Paul's) sticks, batter dipped, french fried	⅓ of pkg.	180
SQUASH, WINTER:		
Acorn, baked	½ cup	56
Hubbard, baked, mashed	½ cup	51
Frozen:		
(Birds Eye)	⅓ of pkg.	43
(Southland) butternut	4-oz. serving	60
STEAK & GREEN PEPPERS, frozen:		
(Green Giant)	9-oz. entree	250
(Swanson)	8½-oz. entree	180
STOCK BASE (French's) beef or chicken	1 tsp.	8
STRAWBERRY:		
Fresh, capped	½ cup	26
Frozen (Birds Eye):		
Halves	⅓ of pkg.	164
Whole	¼ of pkg.	89
Whole, quick thaw	½ of pkg.	125
STRAWBERRY DRINK (Hi-C):		
Canned	6 fl. oz.	89
*Mix	6 fl. oz.	68
STRAWBERRY KRISPIES, cereal (Kellogg's)	¾ cup	110
STRAWBERRY NECTAR, canned (Libby's)	6 fl. oz.	60
STRAWBERRY PRESERVE OR JAM:		
Sweetened:		
(Smucker's)	1 T.	53
(Welch's)	1 T.	52
Dietetic or low calorie:		
(Dia-Mel; Louis Sherry)	1 T.	6
(Diet Delight)	1 T.	12
(Featherweight) calorie reduced	1 T.	16
STUFFING MIX:		
*Beef, *Stove Top*	½ cup	181
*Chicken, *Stove Top*	½ cup	178
*Cornbread, *Stove Top*	½ cup	174
Cube or herb seasoned (Pepperidge Farm)	1 oz.	110
*Pork, *Stove Top*	½ cup	176
White bread (Mrs. Cubbison's)	1 oz.	101

Food and Description	Measure or Quantity	Calories
STURGEON, smoked	4-oz. serving	169
SUCCOTASH:		
Canned:		
(Libby's) cream style	½ cup	111
(Stokely-Van Camp)	½ cup	85
Frozen (Birds Eye)	⅓ of pkg.	104
SUGAR:		
Brown	1 T.	48
Confectioners'	1 T.	30
Granulated	1 T.	46
Maple	1¾" × 1¼" × ½" piece	104
SUGAR CORN POPS, cereal (Kellogg's)	1 cup	110
SUGAR CRISP, cereal (Post)	⅞ cup	112
SUGAR PUFFS, cereal (Malt-O-Meal)	⅞ cup	110
SUGAR SMACKS, cereal (Kellogg's)	¾ cup	110
SUGAR SUBSTITUTE:		
(Estee)	1 tsp.	12
(Featherweight)	3 drops	0
Sprinkle Sweet (Pillsbury)	1 tsp.	2
Sweet'n-it (Dia-Mel) liquid	5 drops	0
SUNFLOWER SEED (Fisher):		
In hull, roasted, salted	1 oz.	86
Hulled, dry roasted, salted	1 oz.	164
Hulled, oil roasted, salted	1 oz.	167
SUZY Q (Hostess):		
Banana	1 piece	240
Chocolate	1 piece	240
SWEETBREADS, calf, braised	4-oz. serving	191
SWEET POTATO:		
Baked, peeled	5" × 1" potato	155
Canned, heavy syrup	4-oz. serving	129
Frozen:		
(Mrs. Paul's) candied, with apples	4-oz. serving	150
(Stouffer's) & apples	5-oz. serving	160
SWISS STEAK, frozen (Swanson) *TV Brand*	10-oz. dinner	350
SWORDFISH, broiled	3" × 3" × ½" steak	218
SYRUP (See also TOPPING):		
Regular:		
Apricot (Smucker's)	1 T.	50
Blackberry (Smucker's)	1 T.	50
Chocolate or chocolate-flavored:		
Bosco	1 T.	55
(Hershey's)	1 T.	52
Corn, *Karo*, dark or light	1 T.	58
Maple, *Karo*, imitation	1 T.	57

Food and Description	Measure or Quantity	Calories
Pancake or waffle:		
(Aunt Jemima)	1 T.	53
Golden Griddle	1 T.	54
Karo	1 T.	58
Log Cabin, regular or buttered	1 T.	56
Mrs. Butterworth's	1 T.	55
Strawberry (Smucker's)	1 T.	50
Dietetic or low calorie:		
Blueberry (Dia-Mel)	1 T.	1
Chocolate or chocolate-flavored		
(Diet Delight)	1 T.	8
Coffee (No-Cal)	1 T.	6
Cola (No-Cal)	1 T.	0
Maple (S&W) *Nutradiet*	1 T.	12
Pancake or waffle:		
(Aunt Jemima)	1 T.	29
(Dia-Mel)	1 T.	1
(Diet Delight)	1 T.	6
(Featherweight)	1 T.	12

T

Food and Description	Measure or Quantity	Calories
TACO:		
*(Ortega)	1 taco	150
*Mix (Durkee)	½ cup	321
Shell (Ortega)	1 shell	50
TAMALE:		
Canned:		
(Hormel beef, *Short Orders*	7½-oz. can	270
Old El Paso, with chili gravy	1 tamale	116
Frozen (Hormel) beef	1 tamale	130
***TANG,** orange, regular	6 fl. oz.	87
TANGERINE OR MANDARIN ORANGE:		
Fresh (Sunkist)	1 large tangerine	39
Canned, solids & liq.:		
Regular pack (Del Monte)	5½-oz. serving	100
Dietetic pack:		
(Diet Delight) juice pack	½ cup	50
(Featherweight) water pack	½ cup	35
(S&W) *Nutradiet*	½ cup	28
TANGERINE DRINK, canned (Hi-C)	6 fl. oz.	90
***TANGERINE JUICE,** from (Minute Maid)	6 fl. oz.	85
TAPIOCA, dry, *Minute,* quick cooking	1 T.	32
TAQUITO, frozen (Van de Kamp's) beef	8-oz. serving	490
TARRAGON (French's)	1 tsp.	5
TASTEEOS, cereal (Ralston Purina)	1¼ cups	110
***TEA:**		
Bag:		
(Lipton):		
Plain or flavored	1 cup	2
Herbal:		
Almond pleasure or cinnamon apple	1 cup	2
Quietly chamomile or toasty spice	1 cup	4
(Sahadi) spearmint	1 cup	4
Instant (Nestea)100%	6 fl. oz.	0
TEAM, cereal	1 cup	110

Food and Description	Measure or Quantity	Calories
TEA MIX, ICED:		
*(Lipton) lemon & sugar flavored	1 cup	60
Nestea, lemon-flavored	1 cup	6
*Dietetic, *Crystal Light*	8 fl. oz.	2
TEQUILA SUNRISE COCKTAIL,		
(Mr. Boston) 12½% alcohol	3 fl. oz.	120
TERIYAKI, frozen (Stouffer's)	10-oz. serving	365
***TEXTURED VEGETABLE PROTEIN,**		
Morningstar Farms:		
Breakfast link	1 link	73
Breakfast patties	1 patty	100
Breakfast strips	1 strip	37
Grillers	1 patty	190
THURINGER:		
(Eckrich) *Smoky Tang*	1-oz. serving	80
(Hormel):		
Beefy	1-oz. serving	100
Old Smokehouse	1-oz. serving	100
(Louis Rich) turkey	1-oz. serving	50
(Oscar Mayer)	.8-oz. slice	72
***TIGER TAILS** (Hostess)	2¼-oz. piece	210
TOASTER CAKE OR PASTRY:		
Pop-Tarts (Kellogg's):		
Regular:		
Blueberry, brown sugar cinnamon or cherry	1 pastry	210
Strawberry	1 pastry	200
Frosted:		
Blueberry, chocolate fudge or strawberry	1 pastry	200
Brown sugar cinnamon, cherry, concord grape or dutch apple	1 pastry	210
Chocolate-vanilla creme	1 pastry	220
Toastes (Howard Johnson) corn	1 slice	112
Toaster Strudel (Pillsbury)	1 slice	190
Toast-R-Cake (Thomas'):		
Blueberry	1 piece	116
Bran	1 piece	113
Corn	1 piece	118
***TOASTIES,** cereal (Post)	1¼ cups	107
***TOASTY O'S,** cereal (Malt-O-Meal)	1¼ cup	110
TOMATO:		
Cherry, whole	4 pieces	14
Regular, whole	1 med. tomato	33
Canned, regular pack, solids & liq.:		
(Contadina) sliced, baby	½ cup	50

Food and Description	Measure or Quantity	Calories
(Del Monte) stewed	4 oz.	37
(Stokely-Van Camp) stewed	½ cup	35
Canned, dietetic pack, solids & liq.:		
(Del Monte) No Salt Added	½ cup	35
(Diet Delight)	½ cup	25
(Featherweight)	½ cup	20
TOMATO JUICE, CANNED:		
Regular pack:		
(Campbell; Libby's)	6-fL.-oz. can	35
(Del Monte)	6-fl.-oz. can	36
Musselman's	6-fl.-oz. can	30
Dietetic pack (Diet Delight; Featherweight)	6 fl. oz.	35
TOMATO JUICE COCKTAIL, canned:		
(Ocean Spray) *Firehouse Jubilee*	6 fl. oz.	44
SnapE-Tom	6 fl. oz.	40
TOMATO PASTE, canned:		
Regular pack:		
(Contadina) Italian	6-oz. serving	210
(Del Monte)	6-oz. can	150
Dietetic (Featherweight) low sodium	6-oz. can	150
TOMATO & PEPPER, HOT CHILI, *Old El Paso,* Jalapeno	1-oz. serving	6
TOMATO, PICKLED (Claussen) green	1 piece	6
TOMATO PUREE, canned:		
Regular (Contadina) heavy	1 cup	100
Dietetic (Featherweight)	1 cup	90
TOMATO SAUCE, canned:		
(Contadina) regular	1 cup	90
(Del Monte):		
Regular or No Salt Added	1 cup	70
Hot	1 cup	80
With tomato bits	1 cup	92
(Hunt's) with cheese	4-oz. serving	70
TOM COLLINS (Mr. Boston) 12½% alcohol	3 fl. oz.	105
TONGUE, beef, braised	4-oz. serving	277
TOPPING:		
Regular:		
Butterscotch (Smucker's)	1 T.	70
Caramel (Smucker's)	1 T.	70
Chocolate fudge (Hershey's)	1 T.	49
Pecans in syrup (Smucker's)	1 T.	65
Pineapple (Smucker's)	1 T.	65
Dietetic, chocolate (Diet Delight)	1 T.	16

Food and Description	Measure or Quantity	Calories
TOPPING, WHIPPED:		
Regular:		
Cool Whip (Birds Eye) dairy	1 T.	16
Lucky Whip, aerosol	1 T.	12
Whip Topping (Rich's)	¼ oz.	20
Dietetic (Featherweight)	1 T.	3
*Mix:		
Regular, *Dream Whip*	1 T.	5
Dietetic (D-Zerta; Estee)	1 T.	4
TOP RAMEN, beef (Nissin Foods)	3-oz. serving	390
TORTILLA (Amigos)	6″ × ⅛″ tortilla	111
TOSTADA, frozen (Van de Kamp's)	8½-oz. serving	530
TOSTADA SHELL (*Old El Paso*)	1 shell	50
TOTAL, cereal	1 cup	110
TRIPE, canned (Libby's)	6-oz. serving	290
TRIPLE SEC LIQUEUR		
(Mr. Boston)	1 fl. oz.	79
TRIX, cereal (General Mills)	1 cup	110
TUNA:		
Canned in oil:		
(Bumble Bee):		
Chunk, light, drained	6½-oz. can	309
Solids, white, drained	7-oz. can	333
(Carnation) solids & liq.	6½-oz. can	427
(Star Kist) solid, white, solids		
& liq.	7-oz. serving	503
Canned in water:		
(Breast O'Chicken)	6½-oz. can	211
(Bumble Bee):		
Chunk, light, solids & liq.	6½-oz. can	234
Solid, white, solids & liq.	7-oz. can	252
(Featherweight) light, chunk	6½-oz. can	210
(Star Kist) light	7-oz. can	220
***TUNA HELPER** (General Mills):		
Country dumplings or noodles cheese	⅕ of pkg.	230
Creamy noodle	⅕ of pkg.	280
TUNA PIE, frozen:		
(Banquet)	8-oz. pie	510
(Morton)	8-oz. pie	370
TUNA SALAD:		
Home recipe	4-oz. serving	193
Canned (Carnation)	¼ of 7½-oz. can	100
TURKEY:		
Barbecued (Louis Rich) breast, half	1 oz.	40
Canned:		
(Hormel) chunk	6¾-oz. serving	230
(Swanson) chunk	2½-oz. serving	120
Packaged:		
(Hormel) breast	1 slice	30

Food and Description	Measure or Quantity	Calories
(Louis Rich):		
Turkey bologna	1-oz. slice	60
Turkey cotto salami	1-oz. slice	50
Turkey ham, chopped	1-oz. slice	45
Turkey pastrami	1-oz. slice	35
(Oscar Mayer) breast	¾-oz. slice	21
Roasted:		
Flesh & skin	4-oz. serving	253
Dark meat	2½" × 1⅛" × ¼" slice	43
Light meat	4" × 2" × ¼" slice	75
Smoked (Louis Rich):		
Drumsticks	1 oz. (without bone)	40
Wing drumettes	1 oz. (without bone)	45
TURKEY DINNER OR ENTREE, FROZEN:		
(Banquet):		
American Favorites	11-oz. dinner	320
Extra Helping	9-oz. dinner	723
(Green Giant)	9-oz. entree	460
(Morton) *Country Table,* sliced	15-oz. dinner	520
(Swanson):		
Regular, with gravy & dressing	9¼-oz. entree	310
(*TV Brand*	11½-oz. dinner	340
(Weight Watchers) sliced, 3-compartment	15¼-oz. meal	380
TURKEY PIE, frozen:		
(Banquet):		
Regular	8-oz. pie	526
Supreme	8-oz. pie	430
(Morton)	8-oz. pie	340
(Stouffer's)	10-oz. pie	460
(Swanson) regular	8-oz. pie	430
TURKEY TETRAZZINI, frozen:		
(Stouffer's)	6-oz. serving	240
(Weight Watchers)	10-oz. pkg.	310
TURNIP GREENS, canned		
(Sunshine) chopped, solids & liq.	½ cup	19
TURNOVER:		
Frozen (Pepperidge Farm):		
Apple or cherry	1 turnover	310
Blueberry, peach or raspberry	1 turnover	320
Refrigerated (Pillsbury)	1 turnover	170
TWINKIE (Hostess):	1 piece	160

V

Food and Description	Measure or Quantity	Calories
VALPOLICELLA WINE (Antinori)	3 fl. oz.	84
VANDERMINT, liqueur	1 fl. oz.	90
VANILLA EXTRACT		
(Virginia Dare)	1 tsp.	10
VEAL, broiled, medium cooked:		
Loin chop	4 oz.	265
Rib, roasted	4 oz.	305
Steak or cutlet, lean & fat	4 oz.	245
VEAL DINNER, FROZEN:		
(Banquet) parmigiana	11-oz. dinner	413
(Swanson) parmigiana:		
Hungry Man	20½-oz. dinner	700
TV Brand	12¼-oz. dinner	450
(Weight Watchers) parmigiana,		
2-compartment	9-oz. meal	250
VEAL STEAK, FROZEN (Hormel):		
Regular	4-oz. serving	130
Breaded	4-oz. serving	240
VEGETABLE BOUILLON (Herb-Ox):		
Cube	1 cube	6
Packet	1 packet	12
VEGETABLE JUICE COCKTAIL:		
Regular, *V-8*	6 fl. oz.	35
Dietetic:		
(S&W) *Nutradiet,* low sodium	6 fl. oz.	35
V-8, low sodium	6 fl. oz.	40
VEGETABLES, MIXED:		
Canned, regular pack:		
(Del Monte) solids & liquids	½ cup	40
(La Choy):		
Chinese	⅓ of 14-oz. pkg.	12
Chop Suey	½ cup	10
(Libby's) solids & liq.	½ cup	40
Canned, dietetic pack		
(Featherweight)	½ cup	40
Frozen:		
(Birds Eye):		
Regular:		
Broccoli, cauliflower &		
carrots in butter sauce	⅓ of pkg.	51

Food and Description	Measure or Quantity	Calories
Carrots, peas & onions, deluxe	⅓ of pkg.	52
Medley, in butter sauce	⅓ of 10-oz. pkg.	62
Mixed, with onion sauce	⅓ of pkg.	103
Farm Fresh:		
Broccoli, cauliflower & carrot strips	⅓ of pkg.	30
Brussels sprouts, cauliflower & carrots	⅓ of pkg.	38
International Style:		
Chinese style	⅓ of pkg.	85
Mexican style	⅓ of pkg.	133
Stir Fry, Chinese style	⅓ of pkg.	36
(Green Giant):		
Regular:		
Broccoli, cauliflower & carrots in cheese sauce	½ cup	60
Corn, broccoli bounty	½ cup	60
Mixed, polybag	½ cup	50
Harvest Fresh	½ cup	60
Harvest Get Togethers:		
Broccoli-cauliflower medley	½ cup	60
Broccoli fanfare	½ cup	80
Japanese style	½ cup	60
(Le Sueur) peas, onions & carrots in butter sauce	½ cup	90
(Southland):		
California blend	⅕ of 16-oz. pkg.	35
Stew	4 oz.	60
VEGETABLES IN PASTRY, FROZEN		
(Pepperidge Farm):		
Asparagus with mornay sauce or broccoli with cheese	3¾ oz.	250
Cauliflower & cheese sauce	3¾ oz.	220
Spinach almondine	3¾ oz.	260
Zucchini provencal	3¾ oz.	210
VEGETABLE STEW, canned *Dinty Moore* (Hormel)	7½-oz. serving	170
"VEGETARIAN FOODS":		
Canned or dry:		
Chicken, fried (Loma Linda) with gravy	1½-oz. piece	109
Chili (Worthington)	½ cup	177
Choplet (Worthington)	1 choplet	50
Dinner cuts (Loma Linda) drained	1 piece	54
Franks, big (Loma Linda)	1.9-oz. frank	100

Food and Description	Measure or Quantity	Calories
Franks, sizzle (Loma Linda)	2.2-oz. frank	167
FriChik (Worthington)	1 piece	75
Granburger (Worthington)	1 oz.	96
Little links (Loma Linda) drained	.8-oz. link	45
Non-meatballs (Worthington)	1 meatball	32
Nuteena (Loma Linda)	½" slice	165
Prime Stakes	1 slice	171
Proteena (Loma Linda)	½" slice	144
Sandwich spread (Loma Linda)	1 T.	24
Savorex (Loma Linda)	1 T.	32
Soyagen, all purpose powder (Loma Linda)	1 T.	48
Soyalac (Loma Linda):		
Concentrate, liquid	1 cup	351
Ready to use	1 cup	166
Soyameat (Wrothington):		
Beef, sliced	1 slice	44
Chicken, diced	1 oz.	40
Soyameal, any kind (Worthington)	1 oz.	120
Stew pack (Loma Linda) drained	1 piece	7
Super links (Worthington)	1 link	110
Swiss steak with gravy (Loma Linda)	1 steak	138
Tender bits (Loma Linda) drained	1 piece	23
Vegelona (Loma Linda)	½" slice	102
Vega-links (Worthington)	1 link	55
Wheat protein	4 oz.	124
Worthington 209	1 slice	58
Frozen:		
Beef pie (Worthington)	1 pie	278
Bologna (Loma Linda)	1 oz.	77
Chicken (Loma Linda)	1 slice	57
Chicken, fried (Loma Linda)	2-oz. serving	188
Chicken pie (Worthington)	1 pie	450
Chic-Ketts (Worthington)	1 oz.	53
Corned beef, sliced (Worthington)	1 slice	32
Fri Pats (Worthington)	1 patty	204
Meatballs (Loma Linda)	1 meatball	46
Meatless salami (Worthington)	1 slice	44
Prosage (Worthington)	1 link	60
Roast beef (Loma Linda)	1 oz.	65
Sausage, breakfast (Loma Linda)	⅓" slice	72
Smoked beef, slices (Worthington)	1 slice	14
Turkey (Loma Linda)	1 oz.	61
Wham, roll (Worthington)	1 sice	36

Food and Description	Measure or Quantity	Calories
VERMOUTH:		
Dry & extra dry (Lejon; Noilly Pratt)	1 fl. oz.	33
Sweet (Lejon; Taylor)	1 fl. oz.	45
VICHY WATER (Schweppes)	Any quantity	0
VINEGAR	1 T.	2

W

Food and Description	Measure or Quantity	Calories
WAFFELOS, cereal (Ralston Purina)	1 cup	110
WAFFLE, frozen:		
(Aunt Jemima) jumbo	1 waffle	86
(Eggo):		
Apple cinnamon	1 waffle	150
Blueberry or strawberry	1 waffle	130
Home style	1 waffle	120
WALNUT, English or Persian		
(Diamond A)	1 cup	679
WALNUT FLAVORING, Black		
(Durkee) imitation	1 tsp.	4
WATER CHESTNUT, canned		
(La Choy) drained	¼ cup	16
WATERCRESS, trimmed	½ cup	3
WATERMELON:		
Wedge	4″ × 8″ wedge	111
Diced	½ cup	21
WELSH RAREBIT:		
Home recipe	1 cup	415
Frozen:		
(Green Giant)	5-oz. serving	219
(Stouffer's)	5-oz. serving	355
WESTERN DINNER, frozen:		
(Banquet) American Favorites	11-oz. dinner	513
(Morton)	11.8-oz. dinner	426
(Swanson) *Hungry Man*	17¾-oz. dinner	820
WHEATENA, cereal	¼ cup	112
WHEAT FLAKES CEREAL		
(Featherweight)	1¼ cups	100
WHEAT GERM, RAW (Elam's)	1 T.	28
WHEAT GERM CEREAL		
(Kretschmer):		
Regular	¼ cup	99
Brown sugar & honey	¼ cup	114
WHEAT HEARTS, cereal		
(General Mills)	1 oz.	110
WHEATIES, cereal	1 cup	110
WHEAT & OATMEAL CEREAL,		
hot (Elam's)	1 oz.	105
WHISKEY SOUR COCKTAIL		
(Mr. Boston)	3 fl. oz.	120

Food and Description	Measure or Quantity	Calories
WHITE CASTLE:		
Bun	.8-oz. bun	65
Cheeseburger (meat & cheese only)	1.54-oz. serving	120
Fish sandwich (fish only, without tartar sauce & bun)	1.5-oz. serving	127
French fries	2.6-oz. serving	225
Hamburger (meat only, no bun)	1.2-oz. serving	95
WHITEFISH, LAKE:		
Baked, stuffed	4 oz.	244
Smoked	4 oz.	176
WIENER WRAP (Pillsbury)	1 piece	60
WILD BERRY DRINK, canned (Hi-C)	6 fl. oz.	88
WINCHELL'S DONUT HOUSE:		
Buttermilk, old fashioned	2-oz. piece	249
Cake, devil's food, iced	2-oz. piece	241
Cinnamon crumb	2-oz. piece	240
Iced, chocolate	2-oz. piece	227
Raised, glazed	1¾-oz. piece	212
WINE, COOKING (Regina):		
Burgundy or sauterne	¼ cup	2
Sherry	¼ cup	20

Y

Food and Description	Measure or Quantity	Calories
YEAST, BAKER's (Fleischmann's):		
Dry, active	¼ oz.	20
Fresh & household, active	.6-oz. cake	15
YOGURT:		
Regular:		
Plain:		
(Bison)	8-oz. container	160
(Colombo):		
Regular	8-oz. container	150
Natural Lite	8-oz. container	110
(Dannon)	8-oz. container	150
(Friendship)	8-oz. container	170
Yoplait	6-oz. container	130
Plain with honey, *Yoplait*,		
Custard Style	6-oz. container	160
Apple:		
(Colombo) spiced	8-oz. container	240
(Dannon) Dutch	8-oz. container	260
Melange	6-oz. container	180
Yoplait	6-oz. container	190
Apple-cinnamon, *Yoplait*,		
Breakfast Yogurt	6-oz. container	240
Apricot (Bison)	8-oz. container	262
Banana:		
(Dannon)	8-oz. container	260
LeShake (Kellogg's)	8-oz. container	170
Banana-Strawberry (Colombo)	8-oz. container	235
Berry (New Country) mixed	8-oz. container	210
Blueberry:		
(Bison):		
Regular	8-oz. container	262
Light	6-oz. container	162
(Dannon)	8-oz. container	260
Melange	6-oz. container	180
(New Country) supreme	8-oz. container	210
(Riche)	6-oz. container	180
(Sweet'n Low)	8-oz. container	150
Yoplait	6-oz. container	190
Boysenberry:		
(Bison)	8-oz. container	262

Food and Description	Measure or Quantity	Calories
(Dannon)	8-oz. container	260
(Sweet 'n Low)	8-oz. container	150
Cherry:		
(Colombo) black	8-oz. container	230
(Dannon)	8-oz. container	260
(Friendship)	8-oz. container	230
Melangé	6-oz. container	180
(Riche)	6-oz. container	180
(Sweet 'n Low)	8-oz. container	150
Yoplait	6-0z. container	150
Cherry-vanilla (Colombo)	8-oz. container	250
Citrus, *Yoplait, Breakfast Yogurt*	6-oz. container	250
Coffee (Colombo; Dannon)	8-oz. container	200
Fruit crunch (New Country)	9-oz. container	210
Guava (Colombo)	8-oz. container	240
Hawaiian salad (New Country)	8-oz. container	210
Honey vanilla (Colombo)	8-oz. container	220
Lemon:		
(Dannon)	8-oz. container	200
(New Country) supreme	8-oz. container	210
(Sweet'n Low)	8-oz. container	150
Yoplait:		
Regular	6-0z. container	190
Custard Style	6-oz. container	180
Orange, *Yoplait*	6-oz. container	190
Orange supreme (New Country)	8-oz. container	210
Orchard, *Yoplait,*		
Breakfast Yogurt	6-oz. container	240
Peach:		
(Bison)	8-oz. container	262
(Dannon)	8-oz. container	260
(Friendship)	8-oz. container	240
(Meadow Gold) sundae style	8-oz. container	260
(New Country) 'n cream	8-oz. container	240
(Riche)	6-oz. container	180
(Sweet'N Low)	8-oz. container	150
Peach melba (Colombo)	8-oz. container	230
Piña colada:		
(Colombo)	8-oz. container	240
(Dannon)	8-oz. container	260
(Friendship)	8-oz. container	230
Pineapple:		
(Bison) light	6-oz. container	162
Melangé	6-oz. container	180
Raspberry:		
(Colombo)	8-oz. container	250
(Dannon) red	8-oz. container	260
Melange	6-oz. container	180

Food and Description	Measure or Quantity	Calories
(Riche)	6-oz. container	180
(Sweet'N Low)	8-oz container	150
Yoplait:		
Regular	6-oz. container	190
Custard Style	6-oz. container	180
Raspberry ripple (New Country)	8-oz. container	240
Strawberry:		
(Colombo)	8-oz. container	230
(Dannon)	8-oz. container	260
(Friendship)	8-oz. container	230
(Meadow Gold)	8-oz. container	270
Melangé	6-oz. container	180
Yoplait	6-oz. container	190
Strawberry-banana (Sweet'N Low)	8-oz. container	190
Strawberry colada (Colombo)	8-oz. container	230
Tropical fruit (Sweet'N Low)	8-oz. container	150
Vanilla:		
(Dannon)	8-oz. container	200
(Friendship)	8-oz. container	210
(New Country) french ripple	8-oz container	240
Yoplait, Custard Style	6-oz. container	180
Frozen, hard:		
Banana, *Danny-in-a-Cup*	8-oz. cup	210
Boysenberry, *Danny-On-A-Stick,* carob coated	2½-fl.-oz. bar	140
Boysenberry swirl (Bison)	¼ of 16-oz. container	116
Cherry vanilla (Bison)	¼ of 16-oz. container	116
Chocolate:		
(Bison)	¼ of 16-oz. container	116
(Colombo) bar, chocolate coated	1 bar	145
(Dannon):		
Danny-in-a-Cup	8-fl.-oz. cup	190
Danny-On-A-Stick, chocolate coated	2½-fl.-oz. bar	130
Chocolate chip (Bison)	¼ of 16-oz. container	116
Chocolate chocolate chip (Colombo)	4-oz. serving	150
Mocha (Colombo) bar	1 bar	80
Piña colada:		
(Colombo)	4-oz. serving	110
(Dannon):		
(Danny-in-a-Cup	8-oz. cup	210
Danny-On-A-Stick	2½-fl.-oz. bar	65

Food and Description	Measure or Quantity	Calories
Raspberry, red (Dannon):		
Danny-in-a-Cup	8-oz. container	210
Danny-On-A-Stick, chocolate coated	2½-fl.-oz. bar	130
Raspberry swirl (Bison)	¼ of 16-oz. container	116
Strawberry:		
(Bison)	¼ of 16-oz. container	116
(Colombo):		
Regular	4-oz. serving	110
Bar	1 bar	80
(Dannon):		
Danny-in-a-Cup	8 fl. oz.	210
Danny-Yo	3½ fl. oz.	110
Vanilla:		
(Bison)	¼ of 16-oz. container	116
(Colombo):		
Regular	4-oz. serving	110
Bar, chocolate coated	1 bar	145
(Dannon):		
Danny-in-a-Cup	8 fl. oz.	180
Danny-On-A-Stick	2½-fl.-oz. bar	65
Danny-Yo	3½-oz. serving	110
Frozen, soft (Colombo)	6-fl.-oz. serving	130

Z

Food and Description	Measure or Quantity	Calories
ZINFANDEL WINE (Inglenook)		
Vintage	3 fl. oz.	59
ZITI, FROZEN (Weight Watchers)	12½-oz. pkg.	342
ZWEIBACK (Gerber: Nabisco)	1 piece	30

Staying Healthy with SIGNET Books